Ensuring a HIPAA-Compliant Informed Consent Process

A Guide for Clinical Research Professionals

Kimberly Irvine
Vice President Operations
Biomedical Research Alliance of New York

Eileen Hilton, M.D.
President and CEO
Biomedical Research Alliance of New York
Professor of Clinical Medicine
Albert Einstein College of Medicine

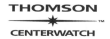

THOMSON
CENTERWATCH™

22 Thomson Place · Boston, MA 02210
Phone (617) 856-5900 · Fax (617) 856-5901
www.centerwatch.com

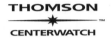

Ensuring a HIPAA-Compliant Informed Consent Process
by Kimberly Irvine & Eileen Hilton, M.D.

Editor	**Publisher**	**Design**
Sara Gambrill	Ken Getz	Paul Gualdoni

ACKNOWLEDGEMENTS

For all of their help in developing this handbook, the authors wish to thank:

Deirdre A. Gutleber Hall, CCRC, CCRA, CIP
Manager, Quality Standards
Pfizer Pharmaceuticals Group

and

Ruth G. Abramson, M.D.
Associate Dean for Research, Mount Sinai School of Medicine
Chairperson, Mount Sinai School of Medicine IRB
Professor of Medicine (Nephrology)

TABLE OF CONTENTS

Table of Contents

Issues addressed include:

- Distinct federal, state and local issues of concern including Health Insurance Portability and Accountability Act of 1996 (HIPAA) regulations
- Tips and suggestions about how to approach consent writing
- The process of informed consent
- Avoiding unnecessary IRB objections
- Avoiding exculpatory language
- Understanding why the investigational site(s) and IRB pick apart sponsor-drafted consent documents and suggestions for preventing this
- Identifying an appropriate contact for subject questions
- Examining whether the consent language places your institution at risk
- Genetic testing consent issues
- Assent—when is it required and sample language
- Sponsor considerations for improving the process
- Glossary of lay terminology

Introduction

Our national health care system relies increasingly on the rapid and wide-spread exchange of printed and electronic patient information. In an effort to protect individuals' rights to control access to and disclosure of private and confidential information, and to ensure continuity of coverage between health insurance plans, the federal government passed The Health Insurance Portability and Accountability Act (HIPAA) in 1996. The HIPAA Privacy Rule, 45 Code of Federal Regulations, Parts 160 and 164, must be fully implemented by April 14, 2003.

The HIPAA Privacy Rule has a far-reaching and significant impact on the clinical research process. It applies to the uses and disclosures of protected health information (PHI) specifically by three types of covered entities: healthcare providers, health plans and healthcare clearinghouses. All clinical investigators, including those who are not otherwise part of these "covered entities," must comply with the Privacy Rule when any of their clinical trials involve investigational treatments. Investigators must also comply with HIPAA if they request PHI from these covered entities.

Protected health information includes study volunteers' names, addresses, phone numbers, fax numbers, email addresses, license plates, Social Security numbers, medical record numbers, health plan beneficiary numbers, data from laboratory work, tissue samples and photographic images. A small percentage of phase I studies of healthy participants may fall outside the scope of HIPAA.

Institutions and independent investigative sites involved with conducting clinical trials must begin their full compliance with the HIPAA Privacy Rule on April 14, 2003. Failure to comply with HIPAA may result in costly civil, or even criminal, sanctions against an institution or independent investigative site.

Obtaining HIPAA Authorization

All study staff must make reasonable efforts to use or disclose only the minimum necessary information on their study subjects. Clinical staff can review a participant's complete medical records and they can share information freely with other clinicians directly involved with that participant's care.

But under the HIPAA Privacy Rule, clinical investigators must also obtain authorization from study subjects in order to use or disclose their identifiable and protected health information. During a clinical research project, study subjects' medical records and their signed consent form will be looked at and copied for scientific and regulatory purposes. Information from the study will be given to the pharmaceutical company sponsoring the research. This information will also be given to the Food and Drug Administration (FDA) and to other regulatory agencies in countries where the drug is being considered for approval.

Unless an exception applies or an institutional review board (IRB) has approved a waiver, clinical investigators may not use or disclose any protected health information without first obtaining signed authorization from study subjects. While the HIPAA Privacy Rule does not require that the authorization form used must first be approved by an IRB prior to reviewing it with study subjects, the Common Rule makes clear that IRBs must be involved wherever human subjects' protection is involved.

The HIPAA Privacy Rule must be implemented within the context of all the other applicable regulations that came before it, and not in isolation. In this context, it is advisable that the IRB review the authorization form. The authorization form must identify the parties that can use and disclose the PHI as well as the parties to whom the PHI may be disclosed. It must also provide study subjects with information related to their rights and recourse, and how their information may be used and disclosed. HIPAA authorization may be incorporated into the body of the informed consent form or it may be provided through the use of a separate authorization document

Consent forms obtained from study subjects prior to April 14, 2003, do not need to be modified until the date of the next continuing review. Clinical investigators are also not required to obtain signed HIPAA authorization forms from study subjects enrolled in trials before April 14, 2003, unless the subjects must be re-consented. This might occur if the protocol is amended or new risks are discovered.

New subjects may be enrolled after the compliance date in trials that were initiated prior to April 14, 2003. In this instance, several options are available. Some organizations plan to use the previously approved consent form and to attach a HIPAA-compliant authorization form. Other organizations plan to rewrite all of their previously approved consent forms in order to comply with HIPAA by the effective date. This approach may be burdensome for larger institutions that are conducting numerous ongoing clinical trials.

From the discussion above, it is clear that complying with the new HIPAA Privacy Rule and obtaining HIPAA authorization from each study subject greatly expands the role and importance of the informed consent process.

This manual is designed to provide practical tips and guidance for creating an informed consent document that complies with the new HIPAA regulations, meets FDA and OHRP guidelines and IRB approval, and is understandable to study subjects.

The manual utilizes the basic framework of a typical informed consent document in order to highlight where required HIPAA elements must be incorporated. Suggested language applicable and compliant with both the Common Rule and HIPAA legislation is provided. In addition, templates for the HIPAA Authorization Form and sample informed consent forms for use in a variety of clinical research studies—genetic testing, tissue banking and assent—are provided. Lastly, as a convenient reference, we include The Final HIPAA Rule in the appendix. Before turning to the consent document framework, we begin with a brief overview of the informed consent process.

The Process of Informed Consent

The informed consent process must take place prior to any involvement of a subject in a research trial. Subjects may voluntarily decide to participate in research only after being fully informed of all associated procedures and their potential risks and benefits. It is the responsibility of the principal investigator to ensure that all information is provided in writing as well as orally and at a comprehension level that can be readily understood.

The regulations anticipate that there will be an oral exchange of information between the investigator and the subject as part of this process. This too must be given in speech understandable to the subject. In addition, if English is not the subject's native language, translated versions (IRB-approved) of the consent document should be available and a translator should be present to confer with the subject. The investigator should encourage and respond to any questions the subject may have. It is important that it be clear to investigators and subjects that there are differences between *obtaining* consent and the informed consent document. The informed consent document should serve as a guide to what will happen during the course of the study.

Thus, informed consent should be regarded as the process that takes place between the subject and the principal investigator or a member of the study staff during which the specifics of the study are discussed. The informed consent discussion should last until both the subject and the person obtaining consent feel confident that the trial has been satisfactorily described and the subject has a reasonable understanding of the consequences of their participation. Potential subjects must be given ample opportunity to consider whether or not they want to participate in a research study. In addition to the informed consent discussion, it is desirable whenever possible to give the prospective participant sufficient time to review the document and discuss it with family and friends. The documentation of the consent process should be in writing and signed and dated by the subject or the subject's legally authorized representative (depending on your state's policy regarding substitute consent).[1]

The individual obtaining consent from the subject should sign and date the document as well. A copy should be given to the subject or the surrogate and the original should be maintained with the investigator's research records. If the subject is an inpatient, some institutions require that a copy of the consent be placed in the medical record.

The Risk of Coercion

People are often vulnerable when discussing health problems with their doctor. They may want to please their caregiver and agree to whatever their physician suggests. It is very important that the investigator minimize the possibility of coercion or undue influence.

Keep It Simple

Consent forms should be written in nonscientific simple terms that research subjects can readily understand. Try to write the consent form at the comprehension level of a sixth grader. This can be challenging for medical professionals. The more familiar one is with medical terminology, the more difficult it becomes to reduce these terms to lay language. A glossary of some commonly used medical terms and some procedures abstracted from the Mount Sinai School of Medicine and the Biomedical Research Alliance of New York's IRB's procedures can be found in the glossary. Other suggestions to improve the readability of the informed consent document may include:

- Prepare the consent document using a 12-point font.
- Avoid run-on sentences and keep sentences and paragraphs short and to the point.
- Use headings to identify new topics and bullets.
- When possible, avoid the use of both the medical term and a lay definition, i.e., insomnia (difficulty sleeping or falling asleep), nausea (upset stomach), anorexia (loss of appetite), as this is more difficult to follow. When in doubt use the lay definition.
- Use proper grammar and punctuation.
- Many IRBs suggest that you use the word "subject" when referring to a research study participant. A patient-doctor relationship is different from a subject-investigator relationship. The word "subject" helps clarify that the discussion is about "research"
- Whenever possible, avoid lengthy consent forms as long forms may affect reading comprehension.

What Is the Goal?

When developing the informed consent document keep in mind the ultimate goal is to provide the potential participant with all the information needed to make an "informed" decision about participation in the research trial.

Defining the Elements of the Informed Consent Form

The U.S. Office for Human Research Protections (OHRP) at 45 CFR 46 and the Code of Federal Regulations (CFR) at 21 CFR 50 and 21 CFR 56 (here and after referred to as The Common Rule) require that certain information be provided to research subjects before they participate in a study.[2] In addition, compliance with HIPAA will be a requirement after April 14, 2003, and is addressed in the sections of the informed consent relating to confidentiality, voluntary participation and statement of consent.

Elements Required by the Common Rule

■ A statement that the study involves research[3]

Example

You are being asked to participate in a research project because you have been diagnosed with high blood pressure.

Common errors and omissions in this section

- Failure to include the reason why the subject is considered a candidate for the study. The statement "You are being invited to participate in a research trial" or something similar is inadequate.
- Use of the word "invite." This should also be replaced with "asked." People are invited to parties not to a research trial.
- Inclusion of the inclusion and exclusion criteria for the study. It is the investigator's responsibility to determine whether or not a subject is eligible for participation. The subject should not have to make this determination.

■ An explanation of the purposes of the research[4]

Example

The primary purpose of this study is to compare the effectiveness and safety of experimental drug, XXX, which has not yet been approved for use by the U.S. Food and Drug Administration (FDA), with that of an FDA-approved drug called YYY.

Common errors and omissions in this section

- Use of terms like "new" instead of "experimental" or "investigational" to describe the status of the study drug. Words like "new" may be perceived as describing a drug that has been "approved" by the FDA. The word "experimental" emphasizes the point that this is research.
- Omission of the definition of an "experimental" drug, for example, "An experimental drug has not yet been approved for use by the U.S. Food and Drug Administration."[5]
- Writing the informed consent document in the "wrong" person. Many but not all IRBs require that the consent form should be written as if the person obtaining consent is presenting it to the subject. The FDA recommends that the consent form be written in the second person ("You/your" instead of "I/my"). Find out your IRB requirements.
- Use of the phrase "You understand." When possible delete words and phrases that reference what the subject is expected to understand. Instead, use clear statements like "Your participation in this study is voluntary" or "You may withdraw from this study at any time without penalty or loss of benefits to which you are otherwise entitled."[6] The consent document must not put subjects in the position of certifying that the information they have received is complete. Avoid using statements such as "You understand all of procedures and risks involved in this study." Instead, try "You have had an opportunity to review this consent form and have all of your questions answered to your satisfaction."
- Neglecting to review the protocol to ensure that the study objectives are reflected in the consent form. Often the rationale for the study is not clearly stated.

■ The expected duration of the subject's participation[7]

Example

Your participation in this study will last 6 weeks.

Common errors and omissions in this section

- Forgetting to inform the subjects of how long their expected participation in the entire study will take.

■ A description of the procedures to be followed[8]

Guidance and Sample Language

- A description of every visit and procedure must be addressed in the consent form including, but not limited to, blood draws,* EKG's, injections, follow-up phone calls, pulmonary function testing, x-ray or any other procedure done in accordance with the protocol. Even completion of questionnaires, diaries or postcards must be included in the consent document. To ensure that all procedures are accounted for, the consent author should compare the procedures listed in the consent form to those described in the protocol.

- If the study requires subjects to be "randomized" or "randomly assigned," this process must be explained to the subject in the consent form. Common phrases that can be used to describe randomization may include "like the flip of a coin" (if the chances are 50/50), "by chance," "like a lottery," "like the roll of the dice" or "picking chances from a hat."

- The dosage of study drug being administered to the subject should be included in this section of the consent form.[9] "If you are randomized to receive drug XXX, you will receive one of the following doses: 300 mg per day, 600 mg per day or 900 mg per day. Your chances of receiving placebo are 1 in 4."

- Is the study double-blinded? This too must be explained. "Neither you nor the investigator will know which treatment you receive. In the event of an emergency, your investigator can determine which drug you are receiving."

- Does the protocol require a washout period? This process must be explained to the patient. "A period of time in which you will be asked not to take your current medication." Is the study open-label, placebo-controlled or evaluator-blinded? These phrases are not lay language and need to be described.

- The consent form should address the duration of individual visits and procedures including questionnaires.

Common errors and omissions in this section

- Listing only "experimental" procedures in the informed consent. All procedures and visits that occur during the protocol must be addressed in the consent. Procedures that are not simply part of

---

* With respect to drawing blood, it is important to include the amount of blood to be drawn. "Approximately 7 tablespoons of blood will be drawn during the course of the study." The amount of blood should be described in measurements of teaspoons or tablespoons (5ml = 1 teaspoon, 15ml = 1 tablespoon). Most subjects have a better idea of the liquid volume of a teaspoon or tablespoon versus a cc (cubic centimeter) or ml (milliliter). Note: a blood count tube is approximately 7ml (1/2 tablespoon) and a serum chemistry tube is approximately 10ml (2 teaspoons).

clinical care but are required as part of the research must still be described in the consent.

- Omission of the length of time associated with procedures, visits, etc.
  - "The quality of life questionnaire will take about 30 minutes to complete."
  - "Study visit 2 will take approximately 1 hour."

■ **Identification of any procedures which are experimental.**[10]

Guidance and Sample Language

- Procedures that are considered experimental must be identified.

  Placing a catheter into the artery to open it up is an alternative to surgery but is considered experimental.

Common errors and omissions in this section

- Failure to distinguish between standard of care and experimental procedures.

■ **A description of any reasonably foreseeable risks or discomforts to the subject**[11]

Guidance and Sample Language

The reported side effects of study drug XXX were generally mild and short-term. The side effects reported most frequently include cough, headache, dizziness and sore throat. These are generally reversible. Rarely, side effects such as swelling of the face, lips, hands or feet, and allergic reaction have occurred. You will be asked to discontinue any current treatment for your high blood pressure, including prescribed medications or herbal therapy, for the duration of the study. If you stop taking your anti-hypertensives, your blood pressure may increase and you may increase your risk of stroke or cardiovascular events…If your condition does not improve or worsens, you should contact the investigator immediately.

You may be given placebo, an inactive substance, during the study. If you receive placebo, your condition may go untreated and may worsen as a result.

The radiation you receive from the chest x-ray is minimal. The more radiation you receive over the course of your life, however, the greater the risk of inducing changes to the cells in your body or of having cancerous tumors. The changes to your body's cells possibly could cause abnormalities or disease in your future offspring. The radiation from this study is not expected to greatly increase these risks, but the exact increase in such risks is not known.

Risks and discomforts associated with drawing blood samples may include pain, bruising, lightheadedness and, on rare occasions, infection.

The study drug must only be taken by the person for whom it has been prescribed and must be kept out of the reach of children and persons of limited capacity to read or understand.

Common errors and omissions in this section

- Omission of the risks of drugs used as part of the research plan, even if they are approved agents. The risks of all drugs used during the study (including placebo) must be disclosed in the consent document.
- Failure to include the risks associated with procedures listed in the protocol. Procedures such as x-rays, placement of an intravenous line, venipuncture, colonoscopy, bronchoscopy and others all carry risks that should be included in the "Risk" section of the informed consent.
- Failure to address the availability of the study drug to the subject once the study is over. Some IRBs require that subjects must be informed whether or not study drug will be available to them once their participation in the study is over.
- Omission of risks associated with stopping or withdrawing from the subject's current medications (washout period).
- Description of risks in medical terms instead of lay terminology (i.e., orthostatic hypotension, respiratory depression, bradycardia and tinnitus).
- Referring to a risk as an "adverse event." It is preferable to use terms such as "side effect" or "bad effect."
- Failure to "cross-check" the "Procedure" section against the "Risk" section to identify omissions in one or both areas.

■ **Pregnancy**

Example

> There may be unforeseen risks to an unborn child associated with your taking Drug XXX. For this reason, you must agree to use a highly effective means of birth control, such as hormonal contraceptives, intrauterine device (IUD), an implantable contraceptive (such as Norplant), an injectable contraceptive (Depo-Provera), a barrier method of contraception (such as a condom or diaphragm with spermicide) or abstinence. You should discuss your methods of birth control with the study doctor. You must notify the investigator if you suspect that you may be pregnant or if you are a male and suspect your partner may be pregnant.[12]

> The effects of Drug XXX on a nursing infant are unknown; if you are breastfeeding, you cannot participate in the study.

Common errors and omissions in this section

- Failure to make reference to males and their partners.
- Not listing the specific methods of birth control that are required by the protocol.
- Not informing the subject that some drugs may interact with hormonal contraceptives rendering them ineffective.

■ **A description of any benefits to the subject or to others which may reasonably be expected from the research[13]**

Example

> Participation in this study may help to improve your condition, but it is also possible that your condition may worsen. There is no guarantee that you will personally benefit by participating in this research study. Your participation in this study may provide information that may help other people who have a similar medical problem in the future."

Common errors and omissions in this section

- Listing payment, free medication and/or close monitoring of "your condition" as benefits of study participation. Such information placed here could be considered coercive and is better located in the "Cost" or "Reimbursement" section of the consent document.
- Omission of a statement such as: "There is no guarantee that you will benefit from study participation."

■ A disclosure of appropriate alternative procedures or courses of treatment, if any, that might be available to the subject[14]

Guidance and Sample Language

> *You do not have to participate in this research study to receive treatment for your condition. You may choose not to be in this study. This will not jeopardize your care in any way. There are other drugs such as XXX, YYY or ZZZ that your doctor can prescribe to treat your condition. The investigator will discuss alternative treatments with you."*

- Alternative medications that may treat the condition under study should be included.
- Subjects must be told that they will be treated for their condition even if they refuse to participate in the research. Subjects should be advised of their options.
- If indicated, inform the subject that there are no alternatives other than not participating. There may be alternative palliative treatments that are not curative. This information should be shared with the subject.
- If the drug used in the study is FDA-approved, subjects should be informed that the study drug is commercially available and that they do not have to participate in the research study to have access to the agent under study.

Common errors and omissions in this section

- Failure to inform subjects that one alternative would be to <u>not</u> participate in the research study.
- Omission of a listing of the other medications or classes of drugs that are available to treat a subject's condition. A statement such as: "Other drugs are available to treat your condition, and the investigator will discuss these alternatives with you" is not very informative. It is often helpful to include brand names if generic names are used.

■ **A statement describing the extent, if any, to which confidentiality of records identifying the subject will be maintained**[15]

The requirements mandated by the Health Insurance Portability and Accountability Act of 1996 (HIPAA) may be incorporated into the body of the consent form or can be addressed in a separate document. (See page 26) Under HIPAA requirements, subjects must authorize the use of their protected health information (PHI). The confidentiality section is appropriate for incorporating some of the required privacy language. Other sections containing sample language relevant to HIPAA include voluntary participation (page 18) and the statement of consent (page 23).[16] In these sections, the HIPAA text will be presented in bold print.

Guidance and Sample Language

Your medical records will be kept as confidential as possible within the limitations of state and federal law. **Federal Privacy Regulations require that you authorize the release of any health information that may reveal your identity. The persons and entities that you are authorizing to use or disclose your individually identifiable health information may include the study doctor, the study staff, the Institution, the Sponsor and (list all applicable parties). In order to analyze the data collected during this research study, all of the health information generated or collected about you during this study** *may be inspected by the study Sponsor or the authorized agents of the sponsor, the FDA, the Department of Health and Human Services (DHHS) agencies, the Institutional Review Board, and governmental agencies in other countries* **(list other parties as appropriate).** *Because of the need to release information to these parties absolute confidentiality cannot be guaranteed.* **Once your personal health information is released it may be redisclosed, at which point your health information will no longer be protected by federal privacy regulations.** *The results of this research may be presented at meetings or in publications; however, your identity will not be disclosed in those presentations. By signing this informed consent form, you are authorizing such access to your medical records.* **This authorization will have no expiration. (Or this authorization will expire on ___/___/___.)**

HIPAA-Required Elements Addressed Here
- Description of information to be used or disclosed
- Persons authorized to use and disclose information
- Persons authorized to receive information
- Purpose of the requested use or disclosure of information
- Redisclosure of information
- Expiration of authorization

Common errors and omissions in this section

- Failure to inform subjects of all the parties that will have access to their medical and study records (sponsors, sponsor representatives, IRB auditors, FDA representatives and other governmental agencies from countries where the study drug may be considered for approval).
- Failure to inform subjects that by signing the consent form they are giving permission for these agencies and representatives to review their records.
- Not clearly stating that absolute confidentiality cannot be guaranteed.

■ **A statement addressing the availability of compensation if injury occurs as a result of study participation**[17]

Guidance and Sample Language

- Sample clauses addressing "Compensation for Injury"

  If you suffer an illness or injury from the study drug or properly performed study procedures, the Sponsor will cover the medical expenses necessary to treat such illness or injury to the extent not covered by insurance or a government program. No other compensation will be offered by the Sponsor or the Institution. By signing this form, you are not waiving any legal right to seek additional compensation through the courts.

  OR

  If you are injured as a result of your participation in this study, immediate, short-term medical care will be made available to you. The costs of such medical care will be billed to you or your insurance company or government program. No other compensation will be offered. You are not waiving any legal rights by signing this form.[18]

- The sponsor will usually provide a clause detailing what costs they will cover in case of illness or injury arising as a result of a subject's participation in the study. This clause should not include statements such as: "Sponsor will not pay for expenses that are attributable to the negligence or misconduct of the Investigator or the Institution." Such language may be considered exculpatory, as it appears to ask subjects to release the sponsor from certain liabilities. Moreover, negligence is a legal term that the subject cannot be expected to understand. Subjects participating in research trials have the same rights as others to seek compensation for an injury, and the consent form should not imply otherwise.
- Other acceptable language: "Only costs in excess of what is paid for by your insurance or other government program will be reimbursed." If applicable, the consent form must clearly state that "No other compensation will be offered by the Sponsor or Institution."
- The "Compensation for Injury" clause should also include some reference to the subject's rights: "You are not giving up any of your legal rights by signing this form," "You are not waiving your legal right to seek additional compensation by signing this form."[19]

The informed consent document must clearly state what form of compensation for injury is available to the subject. If no compensation is available, plainly say so. There is no requirement to discuss compensation that is not available.

Common errors and omissions in this section

- Use of exculpatory language. For example: "No compensation is available," "You will be responsible," or "The sponsor will not be responsible."
- Omission of the entire section. If compensation for injury is unavailable, the section should still be included in the document. Note: If the research is deemed minimal risk, there is no requirement to include compensation for injury language, but many institutions/sponsors/IRBs still include the section.
- Use of complex legal terminology.
- Failure to include a statement explaining that the subject is not waiving any legal rights. Statements made with regard to subjects' rights are sometimes ambiguous. Often we will see the following language in the consent, "You are not waiving any of your rights as a research subject by signing this consent form." This sentence may lead a subject to believe that as a research subject his/her rights differ from the rights of someone not participating in a research study.

■ **An explanation of whom to contact with questions about the research study, research-related injuries or research subjects' rights**[20]

Example

> *If you have any questions concerning your participation in this study, or if you feel you have experienced a research-related injury or a reaction to the study medication you should contact:*
>
> *Dr. Mary Smith at (###) ###-####, the Principal Investigator*
>
> *If you have any questions about your rights as a research subject, you may contact:*
>
> *The Institutional Review Board at (###) ###-#### "*

The consent form must indicate whom subjects should contact if they have any questions about the study, their rights as a research subject or if they think they have suffered an injury as a result of participating in the study.

Common errors and omissions in this section

■ Incorrect phone numbers. One wrong digit may result in a subject's being unable to reach help when he or she has questions or side effects.

■ **A statement indicating that participation is voluntary, refusal to participate will involve no penalty or loss of benefits to which the subject is otherwise entitled, and the subject may discontinue participation at any time without penalty or loss of benefits to which the subject is otherwise entitled**[21]

This is another section of the consent form where HIPAA-related language might be incorporated in the body of the consent.

Guidance and Sample Language

> *Your participation in this research study is voluntary. You have the right to decline participation or to withdraw from this study at any time. This will in no way affect your current or future medical care."*

> *You may also revoke the authorization to use or disclose personal information about your health. If you choose to withdraw your authorization, you must notify the study doctor in writing. The study doctor's mailing address is _____. The study doctor will still be able to use the information collected about you prior to your withdrawal from the study. Information that has already been sent to the study sponsor cannot be withdrawn.**

HIPAA-Required Element Addressed Here
- Right to withdraw authorization

- Subjects must know that their participation in a study is completely voluntary and that they can choose to withdraw from the study at any time without penalty or loss of benefits to which they would otherwise be entitled.[22] If a subject withdraws, he or she should not be jeopardizing his/her relationship with the investigator or the subject's physician, if different.
- **Subjects must also be informed that they can withdraw their authorization to allow the release of any of their individually identifiable health information. However, information that has already been disclosed cannot be withdrawn. It is also important to emphasize that this request must be in writing to the principal investigator.**

Six Elements of the Informed Consent Form Recommended by ICH

The Code of Federal Regulations refers to the remaining six elements listed in this guide as "additional" elements of informed consent to be included when appropriate. The International Conference on Harmonisation (ICH) recommends that these elements be included in all consent forms.

■ **A statement that the particular treatment or procedure may involve risks to the subject that are currently unforeseeable**

Example

> *There may be risks or side effects related to the study drug that are unknown at this time. You will be notified of any signifi-*

---

* If your Institution, Institutional Review Board, or Privacy Board requires the use of a separate authorization form (see page 26) you do not need to include this paragraph in the consent form.

cant new findings that become known that may affect your willingness to continue in the study.[23]

Common errors and omissions in this section

- Failure to include this section in the consent form.

■ **Anticipated circumstances under which the subject's participation may be terminated by the investigator without regard to the subject's consent**[24]

Example

Your participation in this study may be discontinued without your consent by the investigator or the sponsoring company if you fail to follow the investigator's instructions. You may also be withdrawn from the study if, in the investigator's or sponsor's opinion, the study drug is ineffective, harmful or has medically unacceptable side effects, or for other reasons at the discretion of the sponsor or investigator. If you are withdrawn from the study, you will be asked to have the appropriate medical tests and follow-up to evaluate your health and safety.

Common errors and omissions in this section

- Inclusion of a vague blanket statement that subjects may be withdrawn from the study at any time. Subjects must be advised of the possible reasons for withdrawal by the investigator or the sponsor.

■ **Any additional costs to the subject that may result from participation in the research**[25]

Guidance and Sample Language

- Subjects must be informed of any additional costs they may incur related to their participation in the study. If there are no additional costs to the subject the consent form must state so. "There will be no additional cost to you for participation in this research trial" and "The study drug will be provided at no cost to you."
- If the subject's insurance is to be billed for procedures and visits that are part of the research, the subject must be so informed.
- If there is reimbursement for subject's travel expenses or any other compensation, the dollar amount should be clearly defined and an explanation of proration, if any, should be made clear: "You will be

reimbursed a maximum of $150 for your participation in this study to help offset the cost of your time and travel to the investigator's office. If your participation in the study ends prior to study completion, you will be reimbursed $25 for each study visit you completed."

- The subject reimbursement should not be excessive as it may be considered coercive. Usually subjects receive between $25 and $50 for each outpatient visit. Unusually long visits or procedures may carry higher reimbursement. Investigators are encouraged to check their IRB's reimbursement guidelines. Ordinarily, subjects would not receive any compensation for inpatient studies unless the participants are admitted to the hospital solely for the research trial or an outpatient follow-up visit is mandatory.

Common errors and omissions in this section:

- Failure to disclose if the reimbursement will be prorated if they do not complete the study.
- Including information in the "Compensation for Injury" section about additional costs to the subject. "Costs" and "Compensation for Injury" should be two separate and distinct sections of the informed consent document.
- Offering excessive subject reimbursement, raising the possibility of coercion.

- **The consequences of a subject's decision to withdraw from the research and procedures for orderly termination of participation by the subject**[26]

Example

If you decide to withdraw from this research study, you must inform the investigator. For safety reasons, you will be asked to return to the clinic for a final study visit.

Common errors and omissions in this section

- Not including a statement instructing subjects who do not finish the study that it may be in their best interest to return to the clinic for a final visit.
- Suggesting that subjects must return for a final visit.

■ **A statement that significant new findings developed during the course of the research, which may relate to the subject's willingness to continue, will be provided to the subject**[27]

Guidance and Sample Language

You will be notified of any significant new findings that may affect your willingness to continue in the study."

■ This statement can usually be found at the end of the "Risks" section.

■ **The approximate number of subjects involved in the study**[28]

Guidance and Sample Language

Approximately 75 subjects will participate in this research study.

■ A statement of this nature may usually be found in one of two sections in the consent form, either the "Introduction" or the "Purpose of the Study."

Common errors and omissions in this section

■ Not referencing the number of subjects expected to participate in the study.

■ **The study treatment and the probability of random assignment to placebo or to treatment arms**[29]

Guidance and Sample Language

■ The chances of receiving study drug vs. placebo should be documented in the consent form, for example, "Your chances of receiving study drug are 50/50."
■ When applicable, this element is typically found in the "Procedures" section of the consent document where the process of randomization is identified.

Common errors and omissions in this section

- Failing to include the subject's chances of receiving study drug versus another agent or agents.
- Inaccurately describing the chances, such as "like the flip of a coin" when the chances are not 50/50.

■ Statement of Consent[30]

This is another section of the consent form where HIPAA-related language might be incorporated into the body of the consent.

Guidance and Sample Language

> *I have read the above description of this research study. I have been informed of the risks and benefits involved, and all my questions have been answered to my satisfaction. By signing this form, I voluntarily consent to participate in the research study."*

> *Unless I authorize the use and disclosure of my personal health information, I cannot participate in this research study. If I refuse to give my authorization, my medical care will not be affected.* *

HIPAA-Required Element Addressed Here
- Right of refusal

- Typically there is a short consent statement at the end of the document where subjects are asked to confirm they have read the consent form, their questions have been answered satisfactorily, they voluntarily agree to participate in the study, they acknowledge that they are not waiving any legal rights and they authorize release of their medical records.
- There should be a statement here that states, "You will receive a copy of this consent form for your records."

---

* If your Institution, Institutional Review Board, or Privacy Board requires the use of a separate authorization form you do not need to include this paragraph in the consent form.

■ Signatures

Guidance and Sample Language

Guidelines as to who must sign the informed consent form may vary depending on your State, IRB and Institutional requirements. Requested signatures may include: the subject or the subject's legally authorized representative, the principal investigator, the person obtaining consent and/or a witness. Federal policy only requires the signature of the subject or the subject's legally authorized representative when using a standard informed consent document. A witness is not required. In addition, there is no requirement that a subject must initial each page of the consent form. A minimal requirement of most IRBs is a signature by the person obtaining the informed consent.

Avoiding Exculpatory Language

The consent form should not contain exculpatory language. Within the context of informed consent, exculpatory language can be defined as words or phrases that ask or appear to ask a subject to waive or give up his/her legal rights. Exculpatory language may also include asking a subject to release the investigator, sponsor, or institution from liability for negligence or willful misconduct. Avoid using statements that require subjects to agree to terms or conditions as they can be construed as being exculpatory (e.g., "I agree that I will not be paid for any research-related injuries.") Stick to accurate statements. "You will not be offered payment for any research-related injuries."

Examples of Exculpatory Language

By agreeing to this use, you should understand that you would give up all claims to personal benefit from commercial or other use of these substances.

I voluntarily and freely donate any and all blood, urine and tissue and hereby relinquish all right, title and interest to said items.

By consenting to participate in this research, I give up any property rights I may have to the bodily fluids or tissue samples obtained in the course of the research.

I waive any possibility of compensation for injuries that I may receive as a result of participation in this research.

Examples of Acceptable Language

Tissue obtained from you in this research may be used to establish a cell line that could be patented and licensed. There are no plans to provide financial compensation to you should this occur.

By consenting to participate, you authorize the use of your bodily fluids and tissue samples for the research described above.

This hospital is not able to offer financial compensation nor absorb the costs of medical treatment should you be injured as a result of participating in this research.

This hospital makes no commitment to provide free medical care or payment for any unfavorable outcomes resulting from participation in this research. Medical services will be offered at the usual charge.[31]

Assent

Although children are not capable of giving legally valid consent, they may be able to assent or dissent from participation. Assent is "knowledgeable agreement" to participate in a research study and should be used whenever the potential subject has sufficient capacity to understand what is happening and to express his or her wishes. The assent process requires that the investigator and the parent(s) discuss with the child what participation in the research study will involve as well as the possible risks and benefits. Federal regulations require that assent be obtained from all subjects capable of assenting unless certain conditions are met. When determining if minors are capable of giving assent, factors such as the age, the maturity, psychological state and medical condition of potential subjects must be considered. If the condition is life threatening and the research presents the prospect of benefit, the IRB may vote that assent be waived.[32] Some organizations allow verbal assent while others require a written document. Below is a sample for those that use the written format.

Sample Assent Form[33]

Authorization for Release of Information

You are being asked to participate in this research study. You have the right to find out what is involved if you participate, and to tell your parent(s) whether you do or do not want to participate.

Your parents have given permission for you to participate in this study.

Dr. _____ and your parent(s) have explained to you the procedures that are involved with the study.

Dr. _____ and your parent(s) have also explained to you the potential discomforts, risks or inconveniences that may be involved if you participate.

Ask the study doctor any questions you have about the study.

You will receive a copy of this consent form.

Check one:
- ☐   I agree to participate in this study.
- ☐   I do not agree to participate in this study

Child's Name	Child's Age
Child's Signature	Date
Witness to the Assent Process*	Date

*Witness must be a third party unrelated to the family or the study

---

[Note that this form is most often used with younger children. Older teens may be able to assent using the consent form if it is appropriately written. Check on your IRB's policy.]

HIPAA Authorization Form

This separate form is necessary when the required privacy language of the Health Insurance Portability and Accountability Act of 1996 (HIPAA) is not incorporated within the body of the consent. If you choose to address this issue within the informed consent, see pages 15, 16, 18, 19 and 23. The

Authorization Form must include the following Required Elements in order to be in compliance with HIPAA legislation.

General Requirements

- The authorization must be written in plain language.
- A copy of the authorization form must be given to the individual.

Core Elements

- A description of the information to be used or disclosed that identifies the information in a specific and meaningful fashion.
- Name or other specific identification of person(s) or class of persons authorized to use or disclose protected health information (PHI)
- Name or other specific identification of person(s) or class of persons authorized to make the requested use or disclosure of the PHI
- A description of each purpose of the requested use or disclosure. The statement "at the request of the individual" may be sufficient if the statement of purpose is not provided.
- An expiration date or expiration event. One may use "end of the research study" or none.
- A signature of the subject and date.

Required Statements

- A statement that subjects have the right to withdraw their authorization at any time but the notification of such withdrawal must be in writing and, if applicable, explanation of the exceptions to the right to revoke.
- A statement informing subjects that once their PHI has been disclosed it is possible that the receiver may redisclose the information. Subjects must know that at this point their personal information is no longer protected by federal privacy regulations informing subjects that they may review and/or copy any PHI that is disclosed.
- A statement that tells subjects they may refuse to sign the authorization and choosing to refuse will not affect their treatment.[34]

Guidance

- Subjects enrolled prior to April 14, 2003, do not have to be reconsented
- All ongoing research projects will require an authorization form or consent modifications at the time of continuing review.
- New subjects enrolled after April 14, 2003, in ongoing research must sign a separate authorization or a revised IRB-approved consent form incorporating HIPAA-compliant language

Sample HIPAA Authorization Form
Customize for Your Practice

Authorization for Release of Information

I voluntarily authorize the use or disclosure of my individually identifiable health information as described below.

Patient name _____ ID Number_____

Persons/organizations providing the information: Person/organizations receiving the information:

_____ _____

_____ _____

Specific description of information (including date(s)): _____

_____

_____

This information is being disclosed for the following purposes: (e.g., screening and recruiting subjects, analyzing research data) _____

_____

_____

I may revoke this authorization at any time by notifying the practice in writing to [insert name and address]. If I do revoke my authorization, any information previously disclosed cannot be withdrawn. Once information about me is disclosed in accordance with this authorization, the recipient may redisclose it and the information may no longer be protected by federal privacy regulations.

I may refuse to sign this authorization form. If I choose not to sign this authorization form, I cannot participate in the research study.

This authorization will expire the date the research study ends. (Other options for expiration include actual date of expiration, occurrence of a particular event, or "none"; the authorization will have no expiration date.)

I will be given a copy of this authorization form.

_____

Signature of subject or subject's legal representative   Date
(Form MUST be completed before signing)

_____

Printed name of subject's representative:

_____

Relationship to the patient:

YOU MAY REFUSE TO SIGN THIS AUTHORIZATION[35, 36]

Protected Health Information (includes any of the following)

- Names
- Social security numbers
- Geographic subdivisions (i.e., address, zip code)
- Medical record numbers
- All dates (i.e., date of birth, admission date)
- Health plan numbers
- Telephone/fax numbers
- E-mail addresses
- Account numbers
- Vehicle identifier/serial numbers
- Certificate/license numbers
- Device identifier/serial numbers
- IP addresses
- URLs
- DNA, tissue samples or any other materials that may contain identifiable characteristics
- Photos
- Biometric identifiers

Sub-Studies

There may be pharmacogenetic studies or other types of sub-studies done in conjunction with the primary study. The same guidelines that apply to the standard informed consent document also apply to consent documents used for sub-studies. In addition, the consent form must address the following:

- Is participation in the main study contingent upon participation in the sub-study?
- How long will the subject's samples be stored?
- If the subject decides to withdraw from the sub-study, will his or her sample be destroyed or returned?
- Will samples be stored for future use? If so, for what purpose?

The IRB must also approve the future use of the sample.

- Is the sample identifiable or non-identifiable? There are risks associated with both. These risks must also be included in the consent form. It is possible that a commercial or marketable product may be developed as a result of the research done with a subject's sample. This is an area of the consent where you may encounter exculpatory language. An exculpatory statement in this section may be similar to: "You voluntarily donate your samples and you give up all claims to personal benefit from any commercial products that may be developed." Also avoid language such as "the sponsor will be the owner of any data or derivative materials generated from the study" as it may be construed as giving the sponsor property rights, thus waiving those of the subject.

■ Instead, include a sentence such as: "It is possible that the sponsor may develop a commercial product as a result of the data that is collected as part of this study, but there are no plans for you to profit financially from such a product should this occur."

Sample Consent Form for Genetic Testing and/or Tissue Banking[37]

Introduction

Include a general description of the test; explain genetic testing and voluntary participation. For example:

You are being asked to provide one additional blood sample (about 4 teaspoonfuls) for the study described below.

You do not have to agree to be in this additional study in order to be in the main study of Drug XXX and Drug YYY.

DNA is the material in your body's cells (genes) that pass on characteristics that are inherited from one generation to the next (like hair and eye color).

DNA will be extracted from your blood sample in a laboratory so that your genetic information can be used to study whether your response to treatment with Drug XXX and any side effects that you may have developed are related to your genetic identity. This area of research is called "pharmacogenetics" because we are striving to understand how genes influence the different responses people have to the same drug. The goal of this research is to find variations in DNA that will help identify persons with (hypertension) that will have the best response to Drug XXX or to identify persons who will have fewer side effects in order to maximize their benefit from Drug XXX.

Statement of purpose

This is an experimental research study designed specifically to evaluate the relationship of your individual DNA to any improvement in your condition seen with Drug XXX or to any side effects that may arise during treatment. This research study is focused on studying the role genes play in (hypertension) and the responses of the subjects to Drug XXX.

Scope of the project

This study is being conducted at approximately 25 research centers and is expected to involve about 92 subjects."

Statement regarding identification of samples

a. For identified samples:

Your sample will be identified by your subject number, not your name. Only the investigator and the sponsor of the study will be able to link your subject number with your name. Neither you nor your doctor will be given the results of the testing [where applicable].

b. For non-identified samples:

Your sample will be given a number that cannot be linked with you. Your sample will be stored with hundreds of other non-identified samples from [name of institution]. Neither you nor your doctor will be given the results of the testing.

Physical Risks

■ For blood draws:

Although the taking of the blood sample causes no serious problems for most people, it can cause some bleeding, bruising, tiredness, dizziness, and/or discomfort at the injection site.

■ For other collection procedures:
— Describe procedure(s) and attendant risks.

Non-physical risks

There is a chance you may be the subject of discrimination if the results of the testing show a genetic disorder. You might be denied a job or promotion, or denied health or life insurance if employers or insurance companies find out. You may experience other forms of discrimination. We will not release any information to anyone without your written permission. However, it is possible that genetic information may be revealed to others through legal means and may affect your ability to obtain insurance or get a job. In cases where parents and children are both tested, tests may reveal the possibility that the father is not the biological parent.

Potential Benefits of Genetic Testing

This study may improve our understanding of the role of genes in (hypertension). Information learned about the gene may increase general knowledge, provide scientists with information about disease and/or eventually lead to improved treatment. There will be no direct benefit to you or your family from participating in this study."

Confidentiality
Same as previously discussed. (See pages 15 and 16)

Statement regarding contact
Same as previously discussed. (See page 18)

Statement regarding subject injury
Same as previously discussed. (See page 16)

Statement regarding copy of consent
Same as previously discussed. (See page 23)

Statement regarding withdrawal

You are free to withdraw from this study at any time without giving up anything you might otherwise be entitled to. Withdrawal will not have any negative effect on your medical care or anything else. The Investigator may also decide to end your participation in the study at any time. You may request that your sample and data relating to it be destroyed at any time, but this will only be possible if the sample and data can be identified.

Statement regarding use and storage of samples

No tests other than those described in this form will be performed on your sample without your permission. Your sample will be destroyed at the end of the testing process, which is estimated to take approximately 20 years.

OR

Statement regarding storage of samples for general research purposes

In addition to the research outlined in this consent form, your stored sample may be used for general research purposes if you allow it. Please tell us which of the following you agree to (initial all that apply):

___ *The sample may be used for any research project. You do not need to contact me if the sample is to be used for other research even if the sample can be identified with me.*

___ *Future studies can be completed without contacting me if all identifying information is removed so that the sample can't be linked to me.*

___ *I must be contacted prior to using my sample for future studies so that I can decide if I want my sample to be included in the study.*

___ *Under no circumstances may my sample be used for future studies.*

Please tell us (by initialing the applicable line) whether you authorize the researchers to contact you in the future:

___ *I authorize the researchers to contact me in the future for research purposes.*

___ *I do not authorize the researchers to contact me in the future for research purposes.*

Statement regarding use of cell lines (where applicable)

The Investigator may want to use your sample to make a cell line, which means that the cells from your sample would be treated in such a way that they may live and divide outside the body, be frozen for storage indefinitely, and be thawed in the future and used for future genetic research. There are no plans to share with you any financial profits that may result from this research.

Please tell us (by initialing the applicable line) whether you authorize the Investigator to use your sample to make a cell line:

___ *I consent to using my sample to make a cell line*

___ *I do not consent to my sample being used for a cell line.*

Statement of Consent:

I have read this consent form and all of my questions have been answered to my satisfaction. I voluntarily consent to be a subject in this research study and to the procedures described in this form. I have been told that there are no plans to share with me any financial profits resulting from the use of my sample. I am not waiving any legal rights by signing this form.

_____

Printed Name of Subject

_____

Subject Signature   *Date*

_____

Signature of Person Obtaining Consent

Sponsor Considerations for Improving the Informed Consent Process

In a proactive effort, sponsors may go beyond providing individual templates for separate studies, which are then edited by investigators to meet local IRB requirements. Recently, some sponsors have been partnering with IRBs to establish "Master Consent Form Templates." IRBs may review and approve in advance sections of the consent form that consistently remain unchanged. This language, once approved, would be used in every consent form submitted by that sponsor. If these uniform elements are incorporated into the consent form, the approval process is faster and more efficient.

Often, sponsors ask to review any revisions that are made to their individual consent templates prior to and after IRB review. If this is the case, sponsors should keep in mind that IRBs adhere to strict submission deadlines and it is important that sponsors return these consent documents as quickly as possible in order to avoid a delay of study startup as a result of waiting for the next scheduled IRB meeting.

Common Problems With Consent Templates Received From a Study Sponsor

- The document is written in technical terms using medical jargon.
- Exculpatory language is incorporated into the document.
- Sponsors may require patient initials, witness and/or investigator's signature, which might be contradictory to the institution's policy.
- Unclear or understated compensation for injury language. The provision or lack of compensation that the investigational site or sponsor will provide in case of injury should be clearly stated.
- Including the inclusion and exclusion criteria from the protocol.

Afterword

HIPAA compliance is a critical new consideration that is having a great impact on the clinical research process for investigative sites and research sponsors. One of the areas most affected by the HIPAA regulations is the informed consent process. This guide has been created to offer clinical research professionals step-by-step guidance in implementing a HIPAA-compliant informed consent process and in writing a HIPAA-compliant, IRB-acceptable informed consent document or HIPAA authorization document. Ultimately, this guide will give research professionals greater confidence in successfully navigating the uncharted waters of the HIPAA regulations and their application in clinical research.

References

1. 21 CFR 50.25, 45 CFR 46.116
2. Ibid
3. Ibid
4. Ibid
5. Biomedical Research Alliance of New York, Standard Operating Procedures, Policy on: Informed Consent
6. Ibid
7. 21 CFR 50.25, 45 CFR 46.116
8. Ibid
9. Biomedical Research Alliance of New York, Standard Operating Procedures, Policy on: Informed Consent
10. 21 CFR 50.25, 45 CFR 46.116
11. Ibid
12. Ibid
13. Ibid
14. Ibid
15. Ibid
16. HIPAA final rule http://www.hhs.gov/ocr/hipaa/finalreg.html Accessed 10/25/2002
17. Ibid
18. Biomedical Research Alliance of New York, Standard Operating Procedures, Policy on: Informed Consent
19. Ibid
20. 21 CFR 50.25, 45 CFR 46.116
21. Ibid
22. Biomedical Research Alliance of New York, Institutional Review Board, Standard Operating Procedures, Policy on: Informed Consent
23. Ibid
24. 21 CFR 50.25, 45 CFR 46.116
25. Ibid
26. 21 CFR 50.25, 45 CFR 46.116
27. Ibid
28. Ibid
29. Ibid
30. Ibid
31. Office for Protection from Research Risks, Exculpatory Language in Informed Consent Documents, November 15, 1996, World Wide Web http://ohrp.osophs.dhhs.gov/humansubjects/guidance/exculp.htm, access date July 9, 2002
32. 45 CFR 46.408A
33. Biomedical Research Alliance of New York, Institutional Review Board Standard Operating Procedures, Policy: Assent
34. Op. Cit. page 16

35. HIPAA Authorization form. World Wide Web: http://www.karenzupko.
    com/Communities/Ortho/HIPAAAuthorizationFormSample.doc;
    Accessed 10/20/2002

36. Human Research Compliance Insider. Brownstone Publishers, Inc.
    November 2002.

37. Biomedical Research Alliance of New York, Institutional Review Board
    Standard Operating Procedures, Policy: Genetic Testing and Tissue
    Banking

Glossary of Lay Terms for Use in Preparing Informed Consent Documents

Absorb   Take up fluids, take into the body

Acidosis   Condition when blood contains more acid than normal

Acuity   Clearness, keenness, especially of vision, hearing

Acute   New, recent, sudden

Adenopathy   Swollen lymph nodes

Adjuvant   Helpful, assisting, aiding

Adjuvant treatment   Added treatment

Adverse Effect   Side effect of a drug that is undesirable; examples include discomfort or harm to an organ or tissue

Allergic Reaction   May include rash, trouble breathing, fever, and/ or diarrhea

Ambulate/-ation/-ory   Walk, able to walk

Anaphylaxis   Serious, potentially life threatening allergic reaction including reduced blood pressure and difficulty breathing

Anemia   Decreased red blood cells; low red blood cell count which can cause tiredness or fatigue

Anesthetic (general)   A drug or agent used to produce unconsciousness and to decrease the feeling of pain; it puts you to sleep to allow surgery

Anesthetic (local)   A drug or agent used to numb an area of your body to permit surgery or biopsy

Angina   Chest pain from too little blood flow to the heart

Angina Pectoris   Chest pain from too little blood flow to the heart

Antecubital   Area inside the elbow

Antibiotic   Drug that kills bacteria and other germs

Antibody   Protein made in the body in response to a foreign substance; attacks the foreign substance and protects you from infection

Anticonvulsant   Drug used to prevent or treat seizures

Antilipidemic   A drug that decreases the level of fat(s) in the blood

Antimicrobial   Drug that kills bacteria and other germs

Antiretroviral   Drug used to treat HIV or other diseases caused by viruses

Antiviral   Drug used to treat diseases caused by viruses

Antitussive   A drug used to reduce coughing

Arrhythmia   Any change from the normal heartbeat (abnormal heartbeat)

Aspiration   Material entering the lungs following vomiting

Assay   Lab test

Assess   To learn about

Asthma A lung disease associated with narrowing of the breathing passages in the lungs

Asymptomatic Without symptoms

Axilla Armpit

Benign Not harmful, usually without serious consequences, but with some exceptions, e.g. benign brain tumor may have serious consequences

B.i.d. Twice a day

Binding/Bound Carried by/stuck together/transported

Bioavailability The portion of a drug that enters the blood – relates to drugs taken by mouth

Blood Profile Series of blood tests

Bolus An amount given all at once

Bone mass/density The amount of calcium in a given amount of bone

Bradyarrhythmias Slow, irregular heartbeats

Bradycardia Slow heartbeat

Bronchoalveolar Lavage Wash out part of the lung with salt water to obtain lung cells for laboratory tests

Bronchoscopy Insertion of a flexible tube through the nose and voice box to examine the inside of the lung

Bronchospasm Narrowing of the breathing passages of the lung causing difficulty breathing and wheezing

Carcinogenic Capable of causing cancer

Carcinoma Type of cancer

Cardiac Refers to the heart

Cardioversion Return of the normal heartbeat by electric shock or drugs

Catheter A tube inserted into the body for withdrawing or introducing fluids (i.e. a Foley Catheter)

Catheter (Indwelling Epidural) A tube placed near the nerves in the spinal cord used to administer anesthesia during an operation

Cerebral Trauma Damage to the brain

Congestive Heart Disease Hardening of the Arteries of the Heart

Chemotherapy Treatment of disease, usually cancer, by drugs

Chronic Continuing for a long time

Clinical Referring to medical care

Clinical Trial An experiment involving patients

Cognitive Tests Tests of thinking abilities

Complete Response Total disappearance of disease

Consolidation Phase Treatment phase intended to make a remission permanent follows induction

Contraindicated Should not be used

Control Health volunteer

Controlled Trial Study in which the experimental treatment or procedure is compared to a standard (control) treatment or procedure

Cooperative Group Association of multiple hospitals and doctors to perform clinical trials together

Coronary Refers to the blood vessels that supply the heart

Coronary Heart Disease Hardening of the arteries of the heart

CT Scan (CAT) (Computerized Tomography) Computerized series of X-Rays

Culture Test for infection or germs that could cause infection

CVA (Cerebrovascular Accident) Stroke

Diastolic Lower number in blood pressure reading

Distal Toward the end, away from the center of the body

Diuretic "Water Pill" or drug that causes an increase in urination

Doppler Sound waves

Double Blind Study in which neither investigators nor subjects know what drug the subject is receiving

Dysplasia Abnormal Cells

Echocardiogram Sound wave test of the heart

Edema Increased fluid in body tissues, swelling

EEG (Electroencephalogram) Recording of the electric waves in the brain

Efficacy Effectiveness; how well something works

Electrocardiogram ECG or EKG, electrical tracing of the heart

Electrolyte Imbalance Imbalance of minerals in the blood (i.e. potassium, sodium)

Emesis Vomiting

Empiric Based on experience

Endoscopic Insertion of a flexible tube with a light to examine an internal part of the body

Enteral Given through the stomach or intestines

Epidemiologic Referring to the study or the distribution and populations of characteristics and diseases

Epidural A tube placed near the nerves in the spinal cord to administer anesthesia during operation

Extravasate To leak outside of a blood vessel

FDA U.S. Food and Drug Administration, the branch of the federal government which approves new drugs

Fibrillation Irregular beat of the heart or other muscle

Gastrointestinal Relating to the stomach and intestines

General Anesthesia A drug or agent used to produce unconsciousness and to decrease the feeling of pain; it puts you to sleep to allow surgery

Glucose A sugar

Gout A disease that causes a painful inflammation of the joints

Hematocrit Amount of red blood cells in the blood

Hematoma A bruise; a black and blue mark

Hemodynamic Measuring Measuring of blood flow

Hemoglobin A substance in the blood that carries oxygen

Hemolysis Breakdown of red blood cells

Heparin Lock A plastic tube filled with blood thinner that is placed in a vein to give injections or take out blood

Hepatic Refers to the liver

Hepatoma Cancer or tumor of the liver

Holter Monitor A portable machine for recording heartbeats over a period of time

Hypercalcemia Increased level of calcium in the blood

Hyperkalemia Increased level of potassium in the blood

Hypernatremia Increased level of sodium in the blood

Hypertension High blood pressure

Hypocalcemia Reduced level of calcium in the blood

Hyponatremia Reduced level of sodium in the blood

Hypotension Low blood pressure

Hypoxemia A decrease of oxygen in the blood

Hypoxia A decrease of oxygen in the blood

Iatrogenic Cause by a physician or by treatment

IDE Investigational Device Exemption; the license to test an unapproved new medical device

Idiopathic A disorder for which the cause is unknown

Illicit Drugs/Substances Illegal drugs

Immune System The system in the body that reacts to foreign or occasionally one's own proteins

Immunoglobulin A substance produced by the body that binds to a foreign substance

Immunosuppressive Drug which reduces the body's immune response, used in transplantation and diseases caused by disordered immunity

Immunotherapy Use of drugs to help the body's immune (protective) system; usually used to destroy cancer cells

IND Investigational New Drug; the license to test an unapproved new drug

Induction Phase Beginning phase or stage of a treatment

Induration Hardening

Infarct Death of tissue because of lack of blood supply

Infusion Introduction of a substance into the body, usually into the blood through a vein

Ingestion Eating; taking by mouth

Intramuscular Into the muscle; within the muscle

Intrathecal Injected into the space around the spinal cord

Intravenous (IV) Injected into a vein

Intravesical In the bladder

Tracheal Intubation   The placement of a tube into the throat (trachea) to assist breathing

Invasive Procedure   Puncture, opening or cutting of the skin

Ischemia   Decreased oxygen in a tissue (usually because of decreased blood flow)

Leukopenia   Low white blood cell count which can increase the possibility of infection

Lipid Content   Fat content in the blood

Local Anesthesia   A drug or agent used to numb an area of your body to permit surgery or biopsy

Localized   Restricted to one area, limited to one area

Lumen   The cavity of an organ or tube (e.g. blood vessel)

Lymphangiography   An x-ray of the lymph nodes or tissues after injection of dye in lymph vessels (e.g. in feet)

Lymphocyte   A type of white blood cell important in immunity and defense against infection

Lymphoma   A cancer of the lymph nodes (or tissues)

Lumbar Puncture   Spinal Tap; Placement of a needle between the bones in the back to remove some of the fluid around the spinal cord

Malaise   A vague feeling of bodily discomfort, feeling bad

Malignancy   Cancer or other progressively enlarging and spreading tumor, usually fatal if not successfully treated

Medulloblastoma   A type of brain tumor

Megaloblastosis   Change in red blood cells

Metabolize   Process of breaking down substances in cells to obtain energy

Metastasis   Spread of cancer cells from one part of the body to another

MI   Myocardial infarction; heart attack

Minimal   Slight

Minimize   Reduce

Monitor   Check on; keep track of; watch carefully

Mobility   Ease of movement

Morbidity   Undesired result or complication

Mortality   Death or death rate

Motility   The ability to move

MRI   Magnetic resonance imaging; body pictures created using magnetic rather than x-ray energy

Mucosa/Mucous Membrane   Moist lining of digestive, respiratory, reproductive and urinary tracts

Myocardial   Referring to the heart

Myocardial Infarction   Heart Attack

Nasogastric Tube   Tube from the nose to the stomach

NCI   National Cancer Institute

Necrosis   Death of tissue

Neonatal Referring to the newborn period
Neoplasia Tumor, may be benign or malignant
Neuroblastoma A cancer of the nerve tissue
Neutropenia Decrease in the main part of the white blood cells
NIH National Institutes of Health
Non-Invasive Not breaking, cutting or entering the skin
Normal Subject Healthy volunteer
Nosocomial Pneumonia Pneumonia acquired in the hospital

Occlusion Closing; obstruction
Oncology The study of tumors or cancer
Ophthalmic Referring to the eye
Optimal Best, most favorable or desirable
Oral Administration By mouth
Orthopedic Referring to the bones
Osteopetrosis Rare bone disorder characterized dense bone
Osteoporosis Softening of the bones
Ovaries Female sex glands

Parenteral Injection of a drug into a vein or into the skin
Patency Condition of being open
Pathogenesis Causative mechanism in disease
Percutaneous Through the skin
Perforation A tear or a hole
Perinatal Referring to the pregnancy and newborn period
Per Os (PO) By mouth
Pharmacokinetics The study of the way the body absorbs, distributes, metabolizes, and gets rid of a drug
Phase I Initial study of a new drug in humans to determine the limits of tolerance and its safety
Phase II Second phase of a study of a new drug intended to obtain initial information
Phase III Large scale trials to confirm and expand information on safety and usefulness of a new drug
Phlebitis Irritation or inflammation of the vein
Placebo A substance with no active medication
Placebo Effect The perception of improvement when a placebo is given
Platelets Small particles in the blood that help with clotting
Post-Operative After surgery
Potentiate Increase or multiply the effect of a drug or toxin by administration of another drug or toxin at the same time
Potentiator An agent that helps another agent work well
Pre-Operative Before surgery
PRN As needed
Prophylaxis A drug given to prevent disease or infection
Prognosis Chances for recovery

Progresses   Worsens, gets worse
Prone   Lying on the stomach
Prospective   Study following patients forward in time
Protocol   Plan of study
Proximal   Closer to the center of the body, away from the end
Pulmonary   Referring to the lungs

Q.d.   Everyday

Radiation Therapy   X-Ray or Cobalt treatment
Random   By chance
Randomization   Chance selection, like flipping a coin
RBC   Red Blood Cell
Recombinant   Formation of new combinations of genes resulting from
   the manipulation of genes in the laboratory
Reconstitution   Putting back together the original parts or elements; For
   drugs: preparation of a drug for administration by adding liquid to a
   dry, powdered drug
Refractory   Not responding to treatment
Regeneration   Regrowth of a structure or of lost tissue
Relapse   The return of a disease
Remission   Disappearance of evidence of cancer or other disease
Renal   Referring to the kidneys
Replicable   Possible to duplicate
Resect   Remove or cut out surgically
Resolve   Go away
Retrospective Study   Study looking back over past experience

Sedation   Giving medicine to make someone sleepy or less anxious
Seizures   Intense uncontrollable movements
Sequelae   A condition following as a consequence of a disease
Sequential   In a row
Serum   Blood
Spirometry/PFT   Measurement of how well you breathe and how well
   your lungs function
Subcutaneous   Under the skin
Supine   Lying on the back
Systolic   Top number in blood pressure reading
Terminate   Stop
Thoracic   Relating to the chest
Thrombocytopenia   A condition in which there is an abnormally small
   amount of platelets in the blood
Thrombosis   Blood clot
Toxicity   An unwanted side effect resulting in injury to a tissue or organ
Toxicology Test   A test for illegal drugs
Transient   Lasting or staying only a short time

Venipuncture   Blood drawing
Vertigo   Dizziness

The Final HIPAA Rule

45 CFR Part 160
General Administrative Requirements

Subpart A—General Provisions

Subpart B—Preemption of State Law

Subpart C—Compliance and Enforcement

Subpart A—General Provisions

§160.101 Statutory basis and purpose. The requirements of this subchapter implement sections 1171 through 1179 of the Social Security Act (the Act), as added by section 262 of Public Law 104-191, and section 264 of Public Law 104-191.

§160.102 Applicability.

(a) Except as otherwise provided, the standards, requirements, and implementation specifications adopted under this subchapter apply to the following entities:

(1) A health plan.

(2) A health care clearinghouse.

(3) A health care provider who transmits any health information in electronic form in connection with a transaction covered by this subchapter. (b) To the extent required under the Social Security Act, 42 U.S.C. 1320a-7c(a)(5), nothing in this subchapter shall be construed to diminish the authority of any Inspector General, including such authority as provided in the Inspector General Act of 1978, as amended (5 U.S.C. App.).

§160.103 Definitions. Except as otherwise provided, the following definitions apply to this subchapter:

Act means the Social Security Act.

ANSI stands for the American National Standards Institute.

Business associate:

(1) Except as provided in paragraph (2) of this definition, business associate means, with respect to a covered entity, a person who:

(i) On behalf of such covered entity or of an organized health care arrangement (as defined in §164.501 of this subchapter) in which the covered entity participates, but other than in the capacity of a member of the workforce of such covered entity or arrangement, performs, or assists in the performance of:

(A) A function or activity involving the use or disclosure of individually identifiable health information, including claims processing or administration, data analysis, processing or administration, utilization review, quality assurance, billing, benefit management, practice management, and repricing; or

(B) Any other function or activity regulated by this subchapter; or

(ii) Provides, other than in the capacity of a member of the workforce of such covered entity, legal, actuarial, accounting, consulting, data aggregation (as defined in §164.501 of this subchapter), management, administrative, accreditation, or financial services to or for such covered entity, or to or for an organized health care arrangement in which the covered entity participates, where the provision of the service involves the disclosure of individually identifiable health information from such covered entity or arrangement, or from another business associate of such covered entity or arrangement, to the person.

(2) A covered entity participating in an organized health care arrangement that performs a function or activity as described by paragraph (1)(i) of this definition for or on behalf of such organized health care arrangement, or that provides a service as described in paragraph (1)(ii) of this definition to or for such organized health care arrangement, does not, simply through the performance of such function or activity or the provision of such service, become a business associate of other covered entities participating in such organized health care arrangement.

(3) A covered entity may be a business associate of another covered entity.

Compliance date means the date by which a covered entity must comply with a standard, implementation specification, requirement, or modification adopted under this subchapter.

Covered entity means:

(1) A health plan.

(2) A health care clearinghouse.

(3) A health care provider who transmits any health information in electronic form in connection with a transaction covered by this subchapter.

EIN stands for the employer identification number assigned by the Internal Revenue Service, U.S. Department of the Treasury. The EIN is the taxpayer identifying number of an individual or other entity (whether or not an employer) assigned under one or the following:

(1) 26 U.S.C. 6011(b), which is the portion of the Internal Revenue Code dealing with identifying the taxpayer in tax returns and statements, or corresponding provisions of prior law.

(2) 26 U.S.C. 6109, which is the portion of the Internal Revenue Code dealing with identifying numbers in tax returns, statements, and other required documents. Employer is defined as it is in 26 U.S.C. 3401(d).

Group health plan (also see definition of health plan in this section) means an employee welfare benefit plan (as defined in section 3(1) of the Employee Retirement Income and Security Act of 1974 (ERISA), 29 U.S.C. 1002(1)), including insured and self-insured plans, to the extent that the plan provides medical care (as defined in section 2791(a)(2) of the Public Health Service Act (PHS Act), 42 U.S.C. 300gg-91(a)(2)), including items and services paid for as medical care, to employees or their dependents directly or through insurance, reimbursement, or otherwise, that:

(1) Has 50 or more participants (as defined in section 3(7) of ERISA, 29 U.S.C. 1002(7)); or

(2) Is administered by an entity other than the employer that established and maintains the plan.

HCFA stands for Health Care Financing Administration within the Department of Health and Human Services. HHS stands for the Department of Health and Human Services.

Health care means care, services, or supplies related to the health of an individual. Health care includes, but is not limited to, the following:

(1) Preventive, diagnostic, therapeutic, rehabilitative, maintenance, or palliative care, and counseling, service, assessment, or procedure with respect to the physical or mental condition, or functional status, of an individual or that affects the structure or function of the body; and

(2) Sale or dispensing of a drug, device, equipment, or other item in accordance with a prescription.

Health care clearinghouse means a public or private entity, including a billing service, repricing company, community health management information system or community health information system, and "value-added" networks and switches, that does either of the following functions:

(1) Processes or facilitates the processing of health information received from another entity in a nonstandard format or containing nonstandard data content into standard data elements or a standard transaction.

(2) Receives a standard transaction from another entity and processes or facilitates the processing of health information into nonstandard format or nonstandard data content for the receiving entity.

Health care provider means a provider of services (as defined in section 1861(u) of the Act, 42 U.S.C. 1395x(u)), a provider of medical or health services (as defined in section 1861(s) of the Act, 42 U.S.C. 1395x(s)), and any other person or organization who furnishes, bills, or is paid for health care in the normal course of business.

Health information means any information, whether oral or recorded in any form or medium, that:

(1) Is created or received by a health care provider, health plan, public health authority, employer, life insurer, school or university, or health care clearinghouse; and

(2) Relates to the past, present, or future physical or mental health or condition of an individual; the provision of health care to an individual; or the past, present, or future payment for the provision of health care to an individual.

Health insurance issuer (as defined in section 2791(b)(2) of the PHS Act, 42 U.S.C. 300gg-91(b)(2) and used in the definition of health plan in this section) means an insurance company, insurance service, or insurance organization (including an HMO) that is licensed to engage in the business of insurance in a State and is subject to State law that regulates insurance. Such term does not include a group health plan.

Health maintenance organization (HMO) (as defined in section 2791(b)(3) of the PHS Act, 42 U.S.C. 300gg-91(b)(3) and used in the definition of health plan in this section) means a federally qualified HMO, an organization recognized as an HMO under State law, or a similar organization regulated for solvency under State law in the same manner and to the same extent as such an HMO.

Health plan means an individual or group plan that provides, or pays the cost of, medical care (as defined in section 2791(a)(2) of the PHS Act, 42 U.S.C. 300gg-91(a)(2)).

(1) Health plan includes the following, singly or in combination:

(i) A group health plan, as defined in this section.

(ii) A health insurance issuer, as defined in this section.

(iii) An HMO, as defined in this section.

(iv) Part A or Part B of the Medicare program under title XVIII of the Act.

(v) The Medicaid program under title XIX of the Act, 42 U.S.C. 1396, et seq.

(vi) An issuer of a Medicare supplemental policy (as defined in section 1882(g)(1) of the Act, 42 U.S.C. 1395ss(g)(1)).

(vii) An issuer of a long-term care policy, excluding a nursing home fixed-indemnity policy.

(viii) An employee welfare benefit plan or any other arrangement that is established or maintained for the purpose of offering or providing health benefits to the employees of two or more employers.

(ix) The health care program for active military personnel under title 10 of the United States Code.

(x) The veterans health care program under 38 U.S.C. chapter 17.

(xi) The Civilian Health and Medical Program of the Uniformed Services (CHAMPUS)(as defined in 10 U.S.C. 1072(4)).

(xii) The Indian Health Service program under the Indian Health Care Improvement Act, 25 U.S.C. 1601, et seq.

(xiii) The Federal Employees Health Benefits Program under 5 U.S.C. 8902, et seq.

(xiv) An approved State child health plan under title XXI of the Act, providing benefits for child health assistance that meet the requirements of section 2103 of the Act, 42 U.S.C. 1397, et seq.

(xv) The Medicare + Choice program under Part C of title XVIII of the Act, 42 U.S.C. 1395w-21 through 1395w-28.

(xvi) A high risk pool that is a mechanism established under State law to provide health insurance coverage or comparable coverage to eligible individuals.

(xvii) Any other individual or group plan, or combination of individual or group plans, that provides or pays for the cost of medical care (as defined in section 2791(a)(2) of the PHS Act, 42 U.S.C. 300gg-91(a)(2)).

(2) Health plan excludes:

(i) Any policy, plan, or program to the extent that it provides, or pays for the cost of, excepted benefits that are listed in section 2791(c)(1) of the PHS Act, 42 U.S.C. 300gg-91(c)(1); and

(ii) A government-funded program (other than one listed in paragraph (1)(i)-(xvi)of this definition):

(A) Whose principal purpose is other than providing, or paying the cost of, health care; or

(B) Whose principal activity is:

(1) The direct provision of health care to persons; or

(2) The making of grants to fund the direct provision of health care to persons.

Implementation specification means specific requirements or instructions for implementing a standard.

Individually identifiable health information is information that is a subset of health information, including demographic information collected from an individual, and:

(1) Is created or received by a health care provider, health plan, employer, or health care clearinghouse; and

(2) Relates to the past, present, or future physical or mental health or condition of an individual; the provision of health care to an individual; or the past, present, or future payment for the provision of health care to an individual; and

(i) That identifies the individual; or

(ii) With respect to which there is a reasonable basis to believe the information can be used to identify the individual.

Modify or *modification* refers to a change adopted by the Secretary, through regulation, to a standard or an implementation specification.
Secretary means the Secretary of Health and Human Services or any other officer or employee of HHS to whom the authority involved has been delegated.

Small health plan means a health plan with annual receipts of $5 million or less. Standard means a rule, condition, or requirement:

(1) Describing the following information for products, systems, services or practices:

(i) Classification of components.

(ii) Specification of materials, performance, or operations; or

(iii) Delineation of procedures; or

(2) With respect to the privacy of individually identifiable health information.

Standard setting organization (SSO) means an organization accredited by the American National Standards Institute that develops and maintains standards for information transactions or data elements, or any other standard that is necessary for, or will facilitate the implementation of, this part.
State refers to one of the following:

(1) For a health plan established or regulated by Federal law, State has the meaning set forth in the applicable section of the United States Code for such health plan.

(2) For all other purposes, State means any of the several States, the District of Columbia, the Commonwealth of Puerto Rico, the Virgin Islands, and Guam.

Trading partner agreement means an agreement related to the exchange of information in electronic transactions, whether the agreement is distinct or part of a larger agreement, between each party to the agreement. (For example, a trading partner agreement may specify, among other things, the duties and responsibilities of each party to the agreement in conducting a standard transaction.)

Transaction means the transmission of information between two parties to carry out financial or administrative activities related to health care. It includes the following types of information transmissions:

(1) Health care claims or equivalent encounter information.

(2) Health care payment and remittance advice.

(3) Coordination of benefits.

(4) Health care claim status.

(5) Enrollment and disenrollment in a health plan.

(6) Eligibility for a health plan.

(7) Health plan premium payments.

(8) Referral certification and authorization.

(9) First report of injury.

(10) Health claims attachments.

(11) Other transactions that the Secretary may prescribe by regulation.

Workforce means employees, volunteers, trainees, and other persons whose conduct, in the performance of work for a covered entity, is under the direct control of such entity, whether or not they are paid by the covered entity.

§ 160.104 Modifications.

(a) Except as provided in paragraph (b) of this section, the Secretary may adopt a modification to a standard or implementation specification adopted under this subchapter no more frequently than once every 12 months.

(b) The Secretary may adopt a modification at any time during the first year after the standard or implementation specification is initially adopted, if the Secretary determines that the modification is necessary to permit compliance with the standard or implementation specification.

(c) The Secretary will establish the compliance date for any standard or implementation specification modified under this section.

(1) The compliance date for a modification is no earlier than 180 days after the effective date of the final rule in which the Secretary adopts the modification.

(2) The Secretary may consider the extent of the modification and the time needed to comply with the modification in determining the compliance date for the modification.

(3) The Secretary may extend the compliance date for small health plans, as the Secretary determines is appropriate.

Subpart B—Preemption of State Law

§ 160.201 Applicability. The provisions of this subpart implement section 1178 of the Act, as added by section 262 of Public Law 104-191.

§ 160.202 Definitions. For purposes of this subpart, the following terms have the following meanings:

Contrary, when used to compare a provision of State law to a standard, requirement, or implementation specification adopted under this subchapter, means:

(1) A covered entity would find it impossible to comply with both the State and federal requirements; or

(2) The provision of State law stands as an obstacle to the accomplishment and execution of the full purposes and objectives of part C of title XI of the Act or section 264 of Pub. L. 104-191, as applicable. More stringent means, in the context of a comparison of a provision of State law and a standard, requirement, or implementation specification adopted under subpart E of part 164 of this subchapter, a State law that meets one or more of the following criteria:

(1) With respect to a use or disclosure, the law prohibits or restricts a use or disclosure in circumstances under which such use or disclosure otherwise would be permitted under this subchapter, except if the disclosure is:

(i) Required by the Secretary in connection with determining whether a covered entity is in compliance with this subchapter; or

(ii) To the individual who is the subject of the individually identifiable health information.

(2) With respect to the rights of an individual, who is the subject of the individually identifiable health information, regarding access to or amendment of individually identifiable health information, permits greater rights of access or amendment, as applicable.

(3) With respect to information to be provided to an individual who is the subject of the individually identifiable health information about a use, a disclosure, rights, and remedies, provides the greater amount of information.

(4) With respect to the form, substance, or the need for express legal permission from an individual, who is the subject of the individually identifiable health information, for use or disclosure of individually identifiable health information, provides requirements that narrow the scope or duration, increase the privacy protections afforded (such as by expanding the criteria for), or reduce the coercive effect of the circumstances surrounding the express legal permission, as applicable.

(5) With respect to recordkeeping or requirements relating to accounting of disclosures, provides for the retention or reporting of more detailed information or for a longer duration.

(6) With respect to any other matter, provides greater privacy protection for the individual who is the subject of the individually identifiable health information. Relates to the privacy of individually identifiable health information means, with respect to a State law, that the State law has the specific purpose of protecting the privacy of health information or affects the privacy of health information in a direct, clear, and substantial way. State law means a constitution, statute, regulation, rule, common law, or other State action having the force and effect of law.

§ 160.203 General rule and exceptions. A standard, requirement, or implementation specification adopted under this subchapter that is contrary to a provision of State law preempts the provision of State law. This general rule applies, except if one or more of the following conditions is met:

(a) A determination is made by the Secretary under §160.204 that the provision of State law:

(1) Is necessary:

(i) To prevent fraud and abuse related to the provision of or payment for health care;

(ii) To ensure appropriate State regulation of insurance and health plans to the extent expressly authorized by statute or regulation;

(iii) For State reporting on health care delivery or costs; or

(iv) For purposes of serving a compelling need related to public health, safety, or welfare, and, if a standard, requirement, or implementation specification under part 164 of this subchapter is at issue, if the Secretary determines that the intrusion into privacy is warranted when balanced against the need to be served; or

(2) Has as its principal purpose the regulation of the manufacture, registration, distribution, dispensing, or other control of any controlled substances (as defined in 21 U.S.C. 802), or that is deemed a controlled substance by State law.

(b) The provision of State law relates to the privacy of individually identifiable health information and is more stringent than a standard, requirement, or implementation specification adopted under subpart E of part 164 of this subchapter.

(c) The provision of State law, including State procedures established under such law, as applicable, provides for the reporting of disease or injury, child abuse, birth, or death, or for the conduct of public health surveillance, investigation, or intervention.

(d) The provision of State law requires a health plan to report, or to provide access to, information for the purpose of management audits, financial audits, program monitoring and evaluation, or the licensure or certification of facilities or individuals.

§ 160.204 Process for requesting exception determinations.

(a) A request to except a provision of State law from preemption under §160.203(a) may be submitted to the Secretary. A request by a State must be submitted through its chief elected official, or his or her designee. The request must be in writing and include the following information:

(1) The State law for which the exception is requested;

(2) The particular standard, requirement, or implementation specification for which the exception is requested;

(3) The part of the standard or other provision that will not be implemented based on the exception or the additional data to be collected based on the exception, as appropriate;

(4) How health care providers, health plans, and other entities would be affected by the exception;

(5) The reasons why the State law should not be preempted by the federal standard, requirement, or implementation specification, including how the State law meets one or more of the criteria at §160.203(a); and

(6) Any other information the Secretary may request in order to make the determination.

(b) Requests for exception under this section must be submitted to the Secretary at an address that will be published in the Federal Register. Until the Secretary's determination is made, the standard, requirement, or implementation specification under this subchapter remains in effect.

(c) The Secretary's determination under this section will be made on the basis of the extent to which the information provided and other factors demonstrate that one or more of the criteria at §160.203(a) has been met.

§ 160.205 Duration of effectiveness of exception determinations. An exception granted under this subpart remains in effect until:

(a) Either the State law or the federal standard, requirement, or implementation specification that provided the basis for the exception is materially changed such that the ground for the exception no longer exists; or

(b) The Secretary revokes the exception, based on a determination that the ground supporting the need for the exception no longer exists.

Subpart C—Compliance and Enforcement

§ 160.300 Applicability. This subpart applies to actions by the Secretary, covered entities, and others with respect to ascertaining the compliance by covered entities with and the enforcement of the applicable requirements of this part 160 and the applicable standards, requirements, and implementation specifications of subpart E of part 164 of this subchapter.

§ 160.302 Definitions. As used in this subpart, terms defined in §164.501 of this subchapter have the same meanings given to them in that section.

§ 160.304 Principles for achieving compliance.

(a) Cooperation. The Secretary will, to the extent practicable, seek the cooperation of covered entities in obtaining compliance with the applicable requirements of this part 160 and the applicable standards, requirements, and implementation specifications of subpart E of part 164 of this subchapter.

(b) Assistance. The Secretary may provide technical assistance to covered entities to help them comply voluntarily with the applicable requirements of this part 160 or the applicable standards, requirements, and implementation specifications of subpart E of part 164 of this subchapter.

§ 160.306 Complaints to the Secretary.

(a) Right to file a complaint. A person who believes a covered entity is not complying with the applicable requirements of this part 160 or the applicable standards, requirements, and implementation specifications of subpart E of part 164 of this subchapter may file a complaint with the Secretary.

(b) Requirements for filing complaints. Complaints under this section must meet the following requirements:

(1) A complaint must be filed in writing, either on paper or electronically.

(2) A complaint must name the entity that is the subject of the complaint and describe the acts or omissions believed to be in violation of the applicable requirements of this part 160 or the applicable standards, requirements, and implementation specifications of subpart E of part 164 of this subchapter.

(3) A complaint must be filed within 180 days of when the complainant knew or should have known that the act or omission complained of occurred, unless this time limit is waived by the Secretary for good cause shown.

(4) The Secretary may prescribe additional procedures for the filing of complaints, as well as the place and manner of filing, by notice in the Federal Register .

(c) Investigation. The Secretary may investigate complaints filed under this section. Such investigation may include a review of the pertinent policies, procedures, or practices of the covered entity and of the circumstances regarding any alleged acts or omissions concerning compliance.

§ 160.308 Compliance reviews. The Secretary may conduct compliance reviews to determine whether covered entities are complying with the applicable requirements of this part 160 and the applicable standards, requirements, and implementation specifications of subpart E of part 164 of this subchapter.

§ 160.310 Responsibilities of covered entities.

(a) Provide records and compliance reports. A covered entity must keep such records and submit such compliance reports, in such time and manner and containing such information, as the Secretary may determine to be necessary to enable the Secretary to ascertain whether the covered entity has complied or is complying with the applicable requirements of this part 160 and the applicable standards, requirements, and implementation specifications of subpart E of part 164 of this subchapter.

(b) Cooperate with complaint investigations and compliance reviews. A covered entity must cooperate with the Secretary, if the Secretary undertakes an investigation or compliance review of the policies, procedures, or practices of a covered entity to determine whether it is complying with the applicable requirements of this part 160 and the standards, requirements, and implementation specifications of subpart E of part 164 of this subchapter.

(c) Permit access to information.

(1) A covered entity must permit access by the Secretary during normal business hours to its facilities, books, records, accounts, and other sources of information, including protected health information, that are pertinent to ascertaining compliance with the applicable requirements of this part 160 and the applicable standards, requirements, and implementation specifications of subpart E of part 164 of this subchapter. If the Secretary determines that exigent circumstances exist, such as when documents may be hidden or destroyed, a covered entity must permit access by the Secretary at any time and without notice.

(2) If any information required of a covered entity under this section is in the exclusive possession of any other agency, institution, or person and the other agency, institution, or person fails or refuses to furnish the information, the covered entity must so certify and set forth what efforts it has made to obtain the information.

(3) Protected health information obtained by the Secretary in connection with an investigation or compliance review under this subpart will not be disclosed by the Secretary, except if necessary for ascertaining or enforcing compliance with the applicable requirements of this part 160 and the applicable standards, requirements, and implementation specifications of subpart E of part 164 of this subchapter, or if otherwise required by law.

§ 160.312 Secretarial action regarding complaints and compliance reviews.

(a) Resolution where noncompliance is indicated.

(1) If an investigation pursuant to §160.306 or a compliance review pursuant to §160.308 indicates a failure to comply, the Secretary will so inform the covered entity and, if the matter arose from a complaint, the complainant, in writing and attempt to resolve the matter by informal means whenever possible.

(2) If the Secretary finds the covered entity is not in compliance and determines that the matter cannot be resolved by informal means, the Secretary may issue to the covered entity and, if the matter arose from a complaint, to the complainant written findings documenting the noncompliance.

(b) Resolution when no violation is found. If, after an investigation or compliance review, the Secretary determines that further action is not warranted, the Secretary will so inform the covered entity and, if the matter arose from a complaint, the complainant in writing.

45 CFR Part 164
Security and Privacy

Subpart A—General Provisions
§164.102 Statutory basis
§164.104 Applicability
§164.106 Relationship to other parts

Subpart E—Privacy of Individually Identifiable Health Information
§164.500 Applicability
§164.501 Definitions
§164.502 Uses and disclosures of protected health information: general rules
§164.504 Uses and disclosures: organizational requirements
§164.506 Uses and disclosures to carry out treatment, payment, or health care operations
§164.508 Uses and disclosures for which an authorization is required
§164.510 Uses and disclosures requiring an opportunity for the individual to agree or to object
§164.512 Uses and disclosures for which an authorization or opportunity to agree or object is not required
§164.514 Other requirements relating to uses & disclosures of protected health information
§164.520 Notice of privacy practices for protected health information
§164.522 Rights to request privacy protection for protected health information
§164.524 Access of individuals to protected health information
§164.526 Amendment of protected health information
§164.528 Accounting of disclosures of protected health information
§164.530 Administrative requirements
§164.532 Transition provisions
§164.534 Compliance dates for initial implementation of the privacy standards

Authority: 42 U.S.C. 1320d-2 and 1320d-4, sec. 264 of Pub. L. No. 104-191, 110 Stat. 2033-2034 (42 U.S.C. 1320d-2(note)). Subpart A—General Provisions

§164.102 Statutory basis. The provisions of this part are adopted pursuant to the Secretary's authority to prescribe standards, requirements, and implementation specifications under part C of title XI of the Act and section 264 of Public Law 104-191.

§164.104 Applicability. Except as otherwise provided, the provisions of this part apply to covered entities: health plans, health care clearinghouses, and health care providers who transmit health information in electronic form in connection with any transaction referred to in section 1173(a)(1) of the Act.

§164.106 Relationship to other parts. In complying with the requirements of this part, covered entities are required to comply with the applicable provisions of parts 160 and 162 of this subchapter. Subpart B-D—[Reserved]

Subpart E—Privacy of Individually Identifiable Health Information

§164.500 Applicability.

(a) Except as otherwise provided herein, the standards, requirements, and implementation specifications of this subpart apply to covered entities with respect to protected health information.

(b) Health care clearinghouses must comply with the standards, requirements, and implementation specifications as follows:

(1) When a health care clearinghouse creates or receives protected health information as a business associate of another covered entity, the clearinghouse must comply with:

(i) Section 164.500 relating to applicability;

(ii) Section 164.501 relating to definitions;

(iii) Section 164.502 relating to uses and disclosures of protected health information, except that a clearinghouse is prohibited from using or disclosing protected health information other than as permitted in the business associate contract under which it created or received the protected health information;

(iv) Section 164.504 relating to the organizational requirements for covered entities, including the designation of health care components of a covered entity;

(v) Section 164.512 relating to uses and disclosures for which individual authorization or an opportunity to agree or object is not required, except that a clearinghouse is prohibited from using or disclosing protected health information other than as permitted in the business associate contract under which it created or received the protected health information;

(vi) Section 164.532 relating to transition requirements; and

(vii) Section 164.534 relating to compliance dates for initial implementation of the privacy standards.

(2) When a health care clearinghouse creates or receives protected health information other than as a business associate of a covered entity, the clearinghouse must comply with all of the standards, requirements, and implementation specifications of this subpart.

(c) The standards, requirements, and implementation specifications of this subpart do not apply to the Department of Defense or to any other federal agency, or non-governmental organization acting on its behalf, when providing health care to overseas foreign national beneficiaries.

§164.501 Definitions. As used in this subpart, the following terms have the following meanings:

Correctional institution means any penal or correctional facility, jail, reformatory, detention center, work farm, halfway house, or residential community program center operated by, or under contract to, the United States, a State, a territory, a political subdivision of a State or territory, or an Indian tribe, for the confinement or rehabilitation of persons charged with or convicted of a criminal offense or other persons held in lawful custody.

Other persons held in lawful custody includes juvenile offenders adjudicated delinquent, aliens detained awaiting deportation, persons committed to mental institutions through the criminal justice system, witnesses, or others awaiting charges or trial.

Covered functions means those functions of a covered entity the performance of which makes the entity a health plan, health care provider, or health care clearinghouse.

Data aggregation means, with respect to protected health information created or received by a business associate in its capacity as the business associate of a covered entity, the combining of such protected health information by the business associate with the protected health information received by the business associate in its capacity as a business associate of another covered entity, to permit data analyses that relate to the health care operations of the respective covered entities.

Designated record set means:

(1) A group of records maintained by or for a covered entity that is:

(i) The medical records and billing records about individuals maintained by or for a covered health care provider;

(ii) The enrollment, payment, claims adjudication, and case or medical management record systems maintained by or for a health plan; or

(iii) Used, in whole or in part, by or for the covered entity to make decisions about individuals.

(2) For purposes of this paragraph, the term record means any item, collection, or grouping of information that includes protected health information and is maintained, collected, used, or disseminated by or for a covered entity.

Direct treatment relationship means a treatment relationship between an individual and a health care provider that is not an indirect treatment relationship.

Disclosure means the release, transfer, provision of access to, or divulging in any other manner of information outside the entity holding the information.

Health care operations means any of the following activities of the covered entity to the extent that the activities are related to covered functions:

(1) Conducting quality assessment and improvement activities, including outcomes evaluation and development of clinical guidelines, provided that the obtaining of generalizable knowledge is not the primary purpose of any studies resulting from such activities; population-based activities relating to improving health or reducing health care costs, protocol development, case management and care coordination, contacting of health care providers and patients with information about treatment alternatives; and related functions that do not include treatment;

(2) Reviewing the competence or qualifications of health care professionals, evaluating practitioner and provider performance, health plan performance, conducting training programs in which students, trainees, or practitioners in areas of health care learn under supervision to practice or improve their skills as health care providers, training of non-health care professionals, accreditation, certification, licensing, or credentialing activities;

(3) Underwriting, premium rating, and other activities relating to the creation, renewal or replacement of a contract of health insurance or health benefits, and ceding, securing, or placing a contract for reinsur-

ance of risk relating to claims for health care (including stop-loss insurance and excess of loss insurance), provided that the requirements of §164.514(g) are met, if applicable;

(4) Conducting or arranging for medical review, legal services, and auditing functions, including fraud and abuse detection and compliance programs;

(5) Business planning and development, such as conducting cost-management and planning-related analyses related to managing and operating the entity, including formulary development and administration, development or improvement of methods of payment or coverage policies; and

(6) Business management and general administrative activities of the entity, including, but not limited to:

(i) Management activities relating to implementation of and compliance with the requirements of this subchapter;

(ii) Customer service, including the provision of data analyses for policy holders, plan sponsors, or other customers, provided that protected health information is not disclosed to such policy holder, plan sponsor, or customer.

(iii) Resolution of internal grievances;

(iv) The sale, transfer, merger, or consolidation of all or part of the covered entity with another covered entity, or an entity that following such activity will become a covered entity and due diligence related to such activity; and

(v) Consistent with the applicable requirements of §164.514, creating de-identified health information or a limited data set, and fundraising for the benefit of the covered entity.

Health oversight agency means an agency or authority of the United States, a State, a territory, a political subdivision of a State or territory, or an Indian tribe, or a person or entity acting under a grant of authority from or contract with such public agency, including the employees or agents of such public agency or its contractors or persons or entities to whom it has granted authority, that is authorized by law to oversee the health care system (whether public or private) or government programs in which health information is necessary to determine eligibility or compliance, or to enforce civil rights laws for which health information is relevant.

Indirect treatment relationship means a relationship between an individual and a health care provider in which:

(1) The health care provider delivers health care to the individual based on the orders of another health care provider; and

(2) The health care provider typically provides services or products, or reports the diagnosis or results associated with the health care, directly to another health care provider, who provides the services or products or reports to the individual.

Individual means the person who is the subject of protected health information.

Inmate means a person incarcerated in or otherwise confined to a correctional institution.

Law enforcement official means an officer or employee of any agency or authority of the United States, a State, a territory, a political subdivision of a State or territory, or an Indian tribe, who is empowered by law to:

(1) Investigate or conduct an official inquiry into a potential violation of law; or

(2) Prosecute or otherwise conduct a criminal, civil, or administrative proceeding arising from an alleged violation of law.

Marketing means:

(1) To make a communication about a product or service that encourages recipients of the communication to purchase or use the product or service, unless the communication is made:

(i) To describe a health-related product or service (or payment for such product or service) that is provided by, or included in a plan of benefits of, the covered entity making the communication, including communications about: the entities participating in a health care provider network or health plan network; replacement of, or enhancements to, a health plan; and health-related products or services available only to a health plan enrollee that add value to, but are not part of, a plan of benefits.

(ii) For treatment of the individual; or

(iii) For case management or care coordination for the individual, or to direct or recommend alternative treatments, therapies, health care providers, or settings of care to the individual.

(2) An arrangement between a covered entity and any other entity whereby the covered entity discloses protected health information to the other entity, in exchange for direct or indirect remuneration, for the other entity or its affiliate to make a communication about its own product or service that encourages recipients of the communication to purchase or use that product or service.

Organized health care arrangement means:

(1) A clinically integrated care setting in which individuals typically receive health care from more than one health care provider;

(2) An organized system of health care in which more than one covered entity participates, and in which the participating covered entities:

(i) Hold themselves out to the public as participating in a joint arrangement; and

(ii) Participate in joint activities that include at least one of the following:

(A) Utilization review, in which health care decisions by participating covered entities are reviewed by other participating covered entities or by a third party on their behalf;

(B) Quality assessment and improvement activities, in which treatment provided by participating covered entities is assessed by other participating covered entities or by a third party on their behalf; or

(C) Payment activities, if the financial risk for delivering health care is shared, in part or in whole, by participating covered entities through the joint arrangement and if protected health information created or received by a covered entity is reviewed by other participating covered entities or by a third party on their behalf for the purpose of administering the sharing of financial risk.

(3) A group health plan and a health insurance issuer or HMO with respect to such group health plan, but only with respect to protected health information created or received by such health insurance issuer or

HMO that relates to individuals who are or who have been participants or beneficiaries in such group health plan;

(4) A group health plan and one or more other group health plans each of which are maintained by the same plan sponsor; or

(5) The group health plans described in paragraph (4) of this definition and health insurance issuers or HMOs with respect to such group health plans, but only with respect to protected health information created or received by such health insurance issuers or HMOs that relates to individuals who are or have been participants or beneficiaries in any of such group health plans.

Payment means:

(1) The activities undertaken by:

(i) A health plan to obtain premiums or to determine or fulfill its responsibility for coverage and provision of benefits under the health plan; or

(ii) A health care provider or health plan to obtain or provide reimbursement for the provision of health care; and

(2) The activities in paragraph (1) of this definition relate to the individual to whom health care is provided and include, but are not limited to:

(i) Determinations of eligibility or coverage (including coordination of benefits or the determination of cost sharing amounts), and adjudication or subrogation of health benefit claims;

(ii) Risk adjusting amounts due based on enrollee health status and demographic characteristics;

(iii) Billing, claims management, collection activities, obtaining payment under a contract for reinsurance (including stop-loss insurance and excess of loss insurance), and related health care data processing;

(iv) Review of health care services with respect to medical necessity, coverage under a health plan, appropriateness of care, or justification of charges;

(v) Utilization review activities, including precertification and preauthorization of services, concurrent and retrospective review of services; and

(vi) Disclosure to consumer reporting agencies of any of the following protected health information relating to collection of premiums or reimbursement:

(A) Name and address;

(B) Date of birth;

(C) Social security number;

(D) Payment history;

(E) Account number; and

(F) Name and address of the health care provider and/or health plan. Plan sponsor is defined as defined at section 3(16)(B) of ERISA, 29 U.S.C. 1002(16)(B).

Protected health information means individually identifiable health information:

(1) Except as provided in paragraph (2) of this definition, that is:

(i) Transmitted by electronic media;

(ii) Maintained in any medium described in the definition of electronic media at §162.103 of this subchapter; or

(iii) Transmitted or maintained in any other form or medium.

(2) Protected health information excludes individually identifiable health information in:

(i) Education records covered by the Family Educational Rights and Privacy Act, as amended, 20 U.S.C. 1232g;

(ii) Records described at 20 U.S.C. 1232g(a)(4)(B)(iv); and

(iii) Employment records held by a covered entity in its role as employer.

Psychotherapy notes means notes recorded (in any medium) by a health care provider who is a mental health professional documenting or analyzing the contents of conversation during a private counseling session or a group, joint, or family counseling session and that are separated from the rest of the individual's medical record. Psychotherapy notes excludes medication prescription and monitoring, counseling session start and stop times, the modalities and frequencies of treatment furnished, results of clinical tests, and any summary of the following items: diagnosis, functional status, the treatment plan, symptoms, prognosis, and progress to date.

Public health authority means an agency or authority of the United States, a State, a territory, a political subdivision of a State or territory, or an Indian tribe, or a person or entity acting under a grant of authority from or contract with such public agency, including the employees or agents of such public agency or its contractors or persons or entities to whom it has granted authority, that is responsible for public health matters as part of its official mandate.

Required by law means a mandate contained in law that compels an entity to make a use or disclosure of protected health information and that is enforceable in a court of law. Required by law includes, but is not limited to, court orders and court-ordered warrants; subpoenas or summons issued by a court, grand jury, a governmental or tribal inspector general, or an administrative body authorized to require the production of information; a civil or an authorized investigative demand; Medicare conditions of participation with respect to health care providers participating in the program; and statutes or regulations that require the production of information, including statutes or regulations that require such information if payment is sought under a government program providing public benefits.

Research means a systematic investigation, including research development, testing, and evaluation, designed to develop or contribute to generalizable knowledge.

Treatment means the provision, coordination, or management of health care and related services by one or more health care providers, including the coordination or management of health care by a health care provider with a third party; consultation between health care providers relating to a patient; or the referral of a patient for health care from one health care provider to another.

Use means, with respect to individually identifiable health information, the sharing, employment, application, utilization, examination, or analysis of such information within an entity that maintains such information.

§164.502 Uses and disclosures of protected health information: general rules.

(a) Standard. A covered entity may not use or disclose protected health information, except as permitted or required by this subpart or by subpart C of part 160 of this subchapter.

(1) Permitted uses and disclosures. A covered entity is permitted to use or disclose protected health information as follows:

(i) To the individual;

(ii) For treatment, payment, or health care operations, as permitted by and in compliance with §164.506;

(iii) Incident to a use or disclosure otherwise permitted or required by this subpart, provided that the covered entity has complied with the applicable requirements of §164.502(b), §164.514(d), and §164.530(c) with respect to such otherwise permitted or required use or disclosure;

(iv) Pursuant to and in compliance with an authorization that complies with §164.508;

(v) Pursuant to an agreement under, or as otherwise permitted by, §164.510; and

(b(vi) As permitted by and in compliance with this section, §164.512, or §164.514(e), (f), or (g).

(2) Required disclosures. A covered entity is required to disclose protected health information:

(i) To an individual, when requested under, and as required by §164.524 or 164.528; and

(ii) When required by the Secretary under subpart C of part 160 of this subchapter to investigate or determine the covered entity's compliance with this subpart.

(b) Standard: minimum necessary.

(1) Minimum necessary applies. When using or disclosing protected health information or when requesting protected health information from another covered entity, a covered entity must make reasonable

efforts to limit protected health information to the minimum necessary to accomplish the intended purpose of the use, disclosure, or request.

(2) Minimum necessary does not apply. This requirement does not apply to:

(i) Disclosures to or requests by a health care provider for treatment;

(ii) Uses or disclosures made to the individual, as permitted under paragraph (a)(1)(i) of this section or as required by paragraph (a)(2)(i) of this section;

(iii) Uses or disclosures made pursuant to an authorization under §164.508;

(iv) Disclosures made to the Secretary in accordance with subpart C of part 160 of this subchapter;

(v) Uses or disclosures that are required by law, as described by §164.512(a); and

(vi) Uses or disclosures that are required for compliance with applicable requirements of this subchapter.

(c) Standard: uses and disclosures of protected health information subject to an agreed upon restriction. A covered entity that has agreed to a restriction pursuant to §164.522(a)(1) may not use or disclose the protected health information covered by the restriction in violation of such restriction, except as otherwise provided in §164.522(a).

(d) Standard: uses and disclosures of de-identified protected health information.

(1) Uses and disclosures to create de-identified information. A covered entity may use protected health information to create information that is not individually identifiable health information or disclose protected health information only to a business associate for such purpose, whether or not the de-identified information is to be used by the covered entity.

(2) Uses and disclosures of de-identified information. Health information that meets the standard and implementation specifications for de-identification under §164.514(a) and (b) is considered not to be individually identifiable health information, i.e., de-identified. The requirements of this subpart do not apply to information that has been

de-identified in accordance with the applicable requirements of §164.514, provided that:

(i) Disclosure of a code or other means of record identification designed to enable coded or otherwise de-identified information to be re-identified constitutes disclosure of protected health information; and

(ii) If de-identified information is re-identified, a covered entity may use or disclose such re-identified information only as permitted or required by this subpart.

(e)(1) Standard: disclosures to business associates.

(i) A covered entity may disclose protected health information to a business associate and may allow a business associate to create or receive protected health information on its behalf, if the covered entity obtains satisfactory assurance that the business associate will appropriately safeguard the information.

(ii) This standard does not apply:

(A) With respect to disclosures by a covered entity to a health care provider concerning the treatment of the individual;

(B) With respect to disclosures by a group health plan or a health insurance issuer or HMO with respect to a group health plan to the plan sponsor, to the extent that the requirements of §164.504(f) apply and are met; or

(C) With respect to uses or disclosures by a health plan that is a government program providing public benefits, if eligibility for, or enrollment in, the health plan is determined by an agency other than the agency administering the health plan, or if the protected health information used to determine enrollment or eligibility in the health plan is collected by an agency other than the agency administering the health plan, and such activity is authorized by law, with respect to the collection and sharing of individually identifiable health information for the performance of such functions by the health plan and the agency other than the agency administering the health plan.

(iii) A covered entity that violates the satisfactory assurances it provided as a business associate of another covered entity will be in noncompliance with the standards, implementation specifications, and requirements of this paragraph and §164.504(e).

(2) Implementation specification: documentation. A covered entity must document the satisfactory assurances required by paragraph (e)(1) of this section through a written contract or other written agreement or arrangement with the business associate that meets the applicable requirements of §164.504(e).

(f) Standard: deceased individuals. A covered entity must comply with the requirements of this subpart with respect to the protected health information of a deceased individual.

(g)(1) Standard: personal representatives. As specified in this paragraph, a covered entity must, except as provided in paragraphs (g)(3) and (g)(5) of this section, treat a personal representative as the individual for purposes of this subchapter.

(2) Implementation specification: adults and emancipated minors. If under applicable law a person has authority to act on behalf of an individual who is an adult or an emancipated minor in making decisions related to health care, a covered entity must treat such person as a personal representative under this subchapter, with respect to protected health information relevant to such personal representation.

(3) Implementation specification: unemancipated minors.

(i) If under applicable law a parent, guardian, or other person acting in loco parentis has authority to act on behalf of an individual who is an unemancipated minor in making decisions related to health care, a covered entity must treat such person as a personal representative under this subchapter, with respect to protected health information relevant to such personal representation, except that such person may not be a personal representative of an unemancipated minor, and the minor has the authority to act as an individual, with respect to protected health information pertaining to a health care service, if:

(A) The minor consents to such health care service; no other consent to such health care service is required by law, regardless of whether the consent of another person has also been obtained; and the minor has not requested that such person be treated as the personal representative;

(B) The minor may lawfully obtain such health care service without the consent of a parent, guardian, or other person acting in loco parentis, and the minor, a court, or another person authorized by law consents to such health care service; or

(C) A parent, guardian, or other person acting in loco parentis assents to an agreement of confidentiality between a covered health care provider and the minor with respect to such health care service.

(ii) Notwithstanding the provisions of paragraph (g)(3)(i) of this section:

(A) If, and to the extent, permitted or required by an applicable provision of State or other law, including applicable case law, a covered entity may disclose, or provide access in accordance with §164.524 to, protected health information about an unemancipated minor to a parent, guardian, or other person acting in loco parentis;

(B) If, and to the extent, prohibited by an applicable provision of State or other law, including applicable case law, a covered entity may not disclose, or provide access in accordance with §164.524 to, protected health information about an unemancipated minor to a parent, guardian, or other person acting in loco parentis; and

(C) Where the parent, guardian, or other person acting in loco parentis, is not the personal representative under paragraph (g)(3)(i)(A), (B), or (C) of this section and where there is no applicable access provision under State or other law, including case law, a covered entity may provide or deny access under §164.524 to a parent, guardian, or other person acting in loco parentis, if such action is consistent with State or other applicable law, provided that such decision must be made by a licensed health care professional, in the exercise of professional judgment.

(4) Implementation specification: deceased individuals. If under applicable law an executor, administrator, or other person has authority to act on behalf of a deceased individual or of the individual's estate, a covered entity must treat such person as a personal representative under this subchapter, with respect to protected health information relevant to such personal representation.

(5) Implementation specification: abuse, neglect, endangerment situations. Notwithstanding a State law or any requirement of this paragraph to the contrary, a covered entity may elect not to treat a person as the personal representative of an individual if:

(i) The covered entity has a reasonable belief that:

(A) The individual has been or may be subjected to domestic violence, abuse, or neglect by such person; or

(B) Treating such person as the personal representative could endanger the individual; and

(ii) The covered entity, in the exercise of professional judgment, decides that it is not in the best interest of the individual to treat the person as the individual's personal representative.

(h) Standard: confidential communications. A covered health care provider or health plan must comply with the applicable requirements of §164.522(b) in communicating protected health information.

(i) Standard: uses and disclosures consistent with notice. A covered entity that is required by §164.520 to have a notice may not use or disclose protected health information in a manner inconsistent with such notice. A covered entity that is required by §164.520(b)(1)(iii) to include a specific statement in its notice if it intends to engage in an activity listed in §164.520(b)(1)(iii)(A)-(C), may not use or disclose protected health information for such activities, unless the required statement is included in the notice.

(j) Standard: disclosures by whistleblowers and workforce member crime victims.

(1) Disclosures by whistleblowers. A covered entity is not considered to have violated the requirements of this subpart if a member of its workforce or a business associate discloses protected health information, provided that:

(i) The workforce member or business associate believes in good faith that the covered entity has engaged in conduct that is unlawful or otherwise violates professional or clinical standards, or that the care, services, or conditions provided by the covered entity potentially endangers one or more patients, workers, or the public; and

(ii) The disclosure is to:

(A) A health oversight agency or public health authority authorized by law to investigate or otherwise oversee the relevant conduct or conditions of the covered entity or to an appropriate health care accreditation organization for the purpose of reporting the allegation of failure to meet professional standards or misconduct by the covered entity; or

(B) An attorney retained by or on behalf of the workforce member or business associate for the purpose of determining the legal options of the workforce member or business associate with regard to the conduct described in paragraph (j)(1)(i) of this section.

(2) *Disclosures by workforce members who are victims of a crime.* A covered entity is not considered to have violated the requirements of this subpart if a member of its workforce who is the victim of a criminal act discloses protected health information to a law enforcement official, provided that:

(i) The protected health information disclosed is about the suspected perpetrator of the criminal act; and

(ii) The protected health information disclosed is limited to the information listed in §164.512(f)(2)(i).

§164.504 Uses and disclosures: organizational requirements.

(a) Definitions. As used in this section:

Common control exists if an entity has the power, directly or indirectly, significantly to influence or direct the actions or policies of another entity.

Common ownership exists if an entity or entities possess an ownership or equity interest of 5 percent or more in another entity. Health care component means a component or combination of components of a hybrid entity designated by the hybrid entity in accordance with paragraph (c)(3)(iii) of this section.

Hybrid entity means a single legal entity:

(1) That is a covered entity;

(2) Whose business activities include both covered and non-covered functions; and

(3) That designates health care components in accordance with paragraph (c)(3)(iii) of this section.

Plan administration functions means administration functions performed by the plan sponsor of a group health plan on behalf of the group health plan and excludes functions performed by the plan sponsor in connection with any other benefit or benefit plan of the plan sponsor.

Summary health information means information, that may be individually identifiable health information, and:

(1) That summarizes the claims history, claims expenses, or type of claims experienced by individuals for whom a plan sponsor has provided health benefits under a group health plan; and

(2) From which the information described at §164.514(b)(2)(i) has been deleted, except that the geographic information described in §164.514(b)(2)(i)(B) need only be aggregated to the level of a five digit zip code.

(b) Standard: health care component. If a covered entity is a hybrid entity, the requirements of this subpart, other than the requirements of this section, apply only to the health care component(s) of the entity, as specified in this section.

(c)(1) Implementation specification: application of other provisions. In applying a provision of this subpart, other than this section, to a hybrid entity:

(i) A reference in such provision to a "covered entity" refers to a health care component of the covered entity;

(ii) A reference in such provision to a "health plan," "covered health care provider," or "health care clearinghouse" refers to a health care component of the covered entity if such health care component performs the functions of a health plan, health care provider, or health care clearinghouse, as applicable; and

(iii) A reference in such provision to "protected health information" refers to protected health information that is created or received by or on behalf of the health care component of the covered entity.

(2) Implementation specifications: safeguard requirements. The covered entity that is a hybrid entity must ensure that a health care component of the entity complies with the applicable requirements of this subpart. In particular, and without limiting this requirement, such covered entity must ensure that:

(i) Its health care component does not disclose protected health information to another component of the covered entity in circumstances in which this subpart would prohibit such disclosure if the health care component and the other component were separate and distinct legal entities;

(ii) A component that is described by paragraph (c)(3)(iii)(B) of this section does not use or disclose protected health information that it creates or receives from or on behalf of the health care component in a way prohibited by this subpart; and

(iii) If a person performs duties for both the health care component in the capacity of a member of the workforce of such component and for another component of the entity in the same capacity with respect to that component, such workforce member must not use or disclose protected health information created or received in the course of or incident to the member's work for the health care component in a way prohibited by this subpart.

(3) Implementation specifications: responsibilities of the covered entity. A covered entity that is a hybrid entity has the following responsibilities:

(i) For purposes of subpart C of part 160 of this subchapter, pertaining to compliance and enforcement, the covered entity has the responsibility to comply with this subpart.

(ii) The covered entity has the responsibility for complying with §164.530(i), pertaining to the implementation of policies and procedures to ensure compliance with this subpart, including the safeguard requirements in paragraph (c)(2) of this section.

(iii) The covered entity is responsible for designating the components that are part of one or more health care components of the covered entity and documenting the designation as required by §164.530(j), provided that, if the covered entity designates a health care component or components, it must include any component that would meet the definition of covered entity if it were a separate legal entity. Health care component(s) also may include a component only to the extent that it performs:

(A) Covered functions; or

(B) Activities that would make such component a business associate of a component that performs covered functions if the two components were separate legal entities.

(d)(1) Standard: affiliated covered entities. Legally separate covered entities that are affiliated may designate themselves as a single covered entity for purposes of this subpart.

(2) Implementation specifications: requirements for designation of an affiliated covered entity.

(i) Legally separate covered entities may designate themselves (including any health care component of such covered entity) as a single affiliated covered entity, for purposes of this subpart, if all of the covered entities designated are under common ownership or control.

(ii) The designation of an affiliated covered entity must be documented and the documentation maintained as required by §164.530(j).

(3) Implementation specifications: safeguard requirements. An affiliated covered entity must ensure that:

(i) The affiliated covered entity's use and disclosure of protected health information comply with the applicable requirements of this subpart; and

(ii) If the affiliated covered entity combines the functions of a health plan, health care provider, or health care clearinghouse, the affiliated covered entity complies with paragraph (g) of this section.

(e)(1) Standard: business associate contracts.

(i) The contract or other arrangement between the covered entity and the business associate required by §164.502(e)(2) must meet the requirements of paragraph (e)(2) or (e)(3) of this section, as applicable.

(ii) A covered entity is not in compliance with the standards in §164.502(e) and paragraph (e) of this section, if the covered entity knew of a pattern of activity or practice of the business associate that constituted a material breach or violation of the business associate's obligation under the contract or other arrangement, unless the covered entity took reasonable steps to cure the breach or end the violation, as applicable, and, if such steps were unsuccessful:

(A) Terminated the contract or arrangement, if feasible; or

(B) If termination is not feasible, reported the problem to the Secretary.

(2) Implementation specifications: business associate contracts. A contract between the covered entity and a business associate must:

(i) Establish the permitted and required uses and disclosures of such information by the business associate. The contract may not authorize the business associate to use or further disclose the information in a manner that would violate the requirements of this subpart, if done by the covered entity, except that:

(A) The contract may permit the business associate to use and disclose protected health information for the proper management and administration of the business associate, as provided in paragraph (e)(4) of this section; and

(B) The contract may permit the business associate to provide data aggregation services relating to the health care operations of the covered entity.

(ii) Provide that the business associate will:

(A) Not use or further disclose the information other than as permitted or required by the contract or as required by law;

(B) Use appropriate safeguards to prevent use or disclosure of the information other than as provided for by its contract;

(C) Report to the covered entity any use or disclosure of the information not provided for by its contract of which it becomes aware;

(D) Ensure that any agents, including a subcontractor, to whom it provides protected health information received from, or created or received by the business associate on behalf of, the covered entity agrees to the same restrictions and conditions that apply to the business associate with respect to such information;

(E) Make available protected health information in accordance with §164.524;

(F) Make available protected health information for amendment and incorporate any amendments to protected health information in accordance with §164.526;

(G) Make available the information required to provide an accounting of disclosures in accordance with §164.528;

(H) Make its internal practices, books, and records relating to the use and disclosure of protected health information received from, or created or received by the business associate on behalf of, the covered entity available to the Secretary for purposes of determining the covered entity's compliance with this subpart; and

(I) At termination of the contract, if feasible, return or destroy all protected health information received from, or created or received by the business associate on behalf of, the covered entity that the business associate still maintains in any form and retain no copies of such information or, if such return or destruction is not feasible, extend the protections of the contract to the information and limit further uses and disclosures to those purposes that make the return or destruction of the information infeasible.

(iii) Authorize termination of the contract by the covered entity, if the covered entity determines that the business associate has violated a material term of the contract.

(3) Implementation specifications: other arrangements.

(i) If a covered entity and its business associate are both governmental entities:

(A) The covered entity may comply with paragraph (e) of this section by entering into a memorandum of understanding with the business associate that contains terms that accomplish the objectives of paragraph (e)(2) of this section.

(B) The covered entity may comply with paragraph (e) of this section, if other law (including regulations adopted by the covered entity or its business associate) contains requirements applicable to the business associate that accomplish the objectives of paragraph (e)(2) of this section.

(ii) If a business associate is required by law to perform a function or activity on behalf of a covered entity or to provide a service described in the definition of business associate in §160.103 of this subchapter to a covered entity, such covered entity may disclose protected health information to the business associate to the extent necessary to comply with the legal mandate without meeting the requirements of this paragraph (e), provided that the covered entity attempts in good faith to obtain satisfactory assurances as required by paragraph (e)(3)(i) of this section, and, if such attempt fails, documents the attempt and the reasons that such assurances cannot be obtained.

(iii) The covered entity may omit from its other arrangements the termination authorization required by paragraph (e)(2)(iii) of this section, if such authorization is inconsistent with the statutory obligations of the covered entity or its business associate.

(4) Implementation specifications: other requirements for contracts and other arrangements.

(i) The contract or other arrangement between the covered entity and the business associate may permit the business associate to use the information received by the business associate in its capacity as a business associate to the covered entity, if necessary:

(A) For the proper management and administration of the business associate; or

(B) To carry out the legal responsibilities of the business associate.

(ii) The contract or other arrangement between the covered entity and the business associate may permit the business associate to disclose the information received by the business associate in its capacity as a business associate for the purposes described in paragraph (e)(4)(i) of this section, if:

(A) The disclosure is required by law; or

(B)(1) The business associate obtains reasonable assurances from the person to whom the information is disclosed that it will be held confidentially and used or further disclosed only as required by law or for the purpose for which it was disclosed to the person; and

(2) The person notifies the business associate of any instances of which it is aware in which the confidentiality of the information has been breached.

(f)(1) Standard: Requirements for group health plans.

(i) Except as provided under paragraph (f)(1)(ii) or (iii) of this section or as otherwise authorized under §164.508, a group health plan, in order to disclose protected health information to the plan sponsor or to provide for or permit the disclosure of protected health information to the plan sponsor by a health insurance issuer or HMO with respect to the group health plan, must ensure that the plan documents restrict uses and disclosures of such information by the plan sponsor consistent with the requirements of this subpart.

(ii) The group health plan, or a health insurance issuer or HMO with respect to the group health plan, may disclose summary health information to the plan sponsor, if the plan sponsor requests the summary health information for the purpose of :

(A) Obtaining premium bids from health plans for providing health insurance coverage under the group health plan; or

(B) Modifying, amending, or terminating the group health plan.

(iii) The group health plan, or a health insurance issuer or HMO with respect to the group health plan, may disclose to the plan sponsor information on whether the individual is participating in the group health plan, or is enrolled in or has disenrolled from a health insurance issuer or HMO offered by the plan.

(2) Implementation specifications: requirements for plan documents. The plan documents of the group health plan must be amended to incorporate provisions to:

(i) Establish the permitted and required uses and disclosures of such information by the plan sponsor, provided that such permitted and required uses and disclosures may not be inconsistent with this subpart.

(ii) Provide that the group health plan will disclose protected health information to the plan sponsor only upon receipt of a certification by the plan sponsor that the plan documents have been amended to incorporate the following provisions and that the plan sponsor agrees to:

(A) Not use or further disclose the information other than as permitted or required by the plan documents or as required by law;

(B) Ensure that any agents, including a subcontractor, to whom it provides protected health information received from the group health plan agree to the same restrictions and conditions that apply to the plan sponsor with respect to such information;

(C) Not use or disclose the information for employment-related actions and decisions or in connection with any other benefit or employee benefit plan of the plan sponsor;

(D) Report to the group health plan any use or disclosure of the information that is inconsistent with the uses or disclosures provided for of which it becomes aware;

(E) Make available protected health information in accordance with §164.524;

(F) Make available protected health information for amendment and incorporate any amendments to protected health information in accordance with §164.526;

(G) Make available the information required to provide an accounting of disclosures in accordance with §164.528;

(H) Make its internal practices, books, and records relating to the use and disclosure of protected health information received from the group health plan available to the Secretary for purposes of determining compliance by the group health plan with this subpart;

(I) If feasible, return or destroy all protected health information received from the group health plan that the sponsor still maintains in any form and retain no copies of such information when no longer needed for the purpose for which disclosure was made, except that, if such return or destruction is not feasible, limit further uses and disclosures to those purposes that make the return or destruction of the information infeasible; and

(J) Ensure that the adequate separation required in paragraph (f)(2)(iii) of this section is established.

(iii) Provide for adequate separation between the group health plan and the plan sponsor. The plan documents must:

(A) Describe those employees or classes of employees or other persons under the control of the plan sponsor to be given access to the protected health information to be disclosed, provided that any employee or person who receives protected health information relating to payment under, health care operations of, or other matters pertaining to the group health plan in the ordinary course of business must be included in such description;

(B) Restrict the access to and use by such employees and other persons described in paragraph (f)(2)(iii)(A) of this section to the plan administration functions that the plan sponsor performs for the group health plan; and

(C) Provide an effective mechanism for resolving any issues of noncompliance by persons described in paragraph (f)(2)(iii)(A) of this section with the plan document provisions required by this paragraph.

(3) Implementation specifications: uses and disclosures. A group health plan may:

(i) Disclose protected health information to a plan sponsor to carry out plan administration functions that the plan sponsor performs only consistent with the provisions of paragraph (f)(2) of this section;

(ii) Not permit a health insurance issuer or HMO with respect to the group health plan to disclose protected health information to the plan sponsor except as permitted by this paragraph;

(iii) Not disclose and may not permit a health insurance issuer or HMO to disclose protected health information to a plan sponsor as otherwise permitted by this paragraph unless a statement required by §164.520(b)(1)(iii)(C) is included in the appropriate notice; and

(iv) Not disclose protected health information to the plan sponsor for the purpose of employment-related actions or decisions or in connection with any other benefit or employee benefit plan of the plan sponsor.

(g) Standard: requirements for a covered entity with multiple covered functions.

(1) A covered entity that performs multiple covered functions that would make the entity any combination of a health plan, a covered health care provider, and a health care clearinghouse, must comply with the standards, requirements, and implementation specifications of this subpart, as applicable to the health plan, health care provider, or health care clearinghouse covered functions performed.

(2) A covered entity that performs multiple covered functions may use or disclose the protected health information of individuals who receive the covered entity's health plan or health care provider services, but not both, only for purposes related to the appropriate function being performed.

§164.506 Uses and disclosures to carry out treatment, payment, or health care operations.

(a) Standard: Permitted uses and disclosures. Except with respect to uses or disclosures that require an authorization under §164.508(a)(2) and (3), a covered entity may use or disclose protected health information for treatment, payment, or health care operations as set forth in paragraph (c) of this section, provided that such use or disclosure is consistent with other applicable requirements of this subpart.

(b) Standard: Consent for uses and disclosures permitted.

(1) A covered entity may obtain consent of the individual to use or disclose protected health information to carry out treatment, payment, or health care operations.

(2) Consent, under paragraph (b) of this section, shall not be effective to permit a use or disclosure of protected health information when an authorization, under §164.508, is required or when another condition must be met for such use or disclosure to be permissible under this subpart.

(c) Implementation specifications: Treatment, payment, or health care operations.

(1) A covered entity may use or disclose protected health information for its own treatment, payment, or health care operations.

(2) A covered entity may disclose protected health information for treatment activities of a health care provider.

(3) A covered entity may disclose protected health information to another covered entity or a health care provider for the payment activities of the entity that receives the information.

(4) A covered entity may disclose protected health information to another covered entity for health care operations activities of the entity that receives the information, if each entity either has or had a relationship with the individual who is the subject of the protected health information being requested, the protected health information pertains to such relationship, and the disclosure is:

(i) For a purpose listed in paragraph (1) or (2) of the definition of health care operations; or

(ii) For the purpose of health care fraud and abuse detection or compliance.

(5) A covered entity that participates in an organized health care arrangement may disclose protected health information about an individual to another covered entity that participates in the organized health care arrangement for any health care operations activities of the organized health care arrangement.

§164.508 Uses and disclosures for which an authorization is required.

(a) Standard: authorizations for uses and disclosures.

(1) Authorization required: general rule. Except as otherwise permitted or required by this subchapter, a covered entity may not use or disclose protected health information without an authorization that is valid under this section. When a covered entity obtains or receives a valid authorization for its use or disclosure of protected health information, such use or disclosure must be consistent with such authorization.

(2) Authorization required: psychotherapy notes. Notwithstanding any provision of this subpart, other than the transition provisions in §164.532, a covered entity must obtain an authorization for any use or disclosure of psychotherapy notes, except:

(i) To carry out the following treatment, payment, or health care operations:

(A) Use by the originator of the psychotherapy notes for treatment;

(B) Use or disclosure by the covered entity for its own training programs in which students, trainees, or practitioners in mental health learn under supervision to practice or improve their skills in group, joint, family, or individual counseling; or

(C) Use or disclosure by the covered entity to defend itself in a legal action or other proceeding brought by the individual; and

(ii) A use or disclosure that is required by §164.502(a)(2)(ii) or permitted by §164.512(a); §164.512(d) with respect to the oversight of the originator of the psychotherapy notes; §164.512(g)(1); or §164.512(j)(1)(i).

(3) Authorization required: Marketing.

(i) Notwithstanding any provision of this subpart, other than the transition provisions in §164.532, a covered entity must obtain an authorization for any use or disclosure of protected health information for marketing, except if the communication is in the form of:

(A) A face-to-face communication made by a covered entity to an individual; or

(B) A promotional gift of nominal value provided by the covered entity.

(ii) If the marketing involves direct or indirect remuneration to the covered entity from a third party, the authorization must state that such remuneration is involved.

(b) Implementation specifications: general requirements.

(1) Valid authorizations.

(i) A valid authorization is a document that meets the requirements in paragraphs (a)(3)(ii), (c)(1), and (c)(2) of this section, as applicable.

(ii) A valid authorization may contain elements or information in addition to the elements required by this section, provided that such additional elements or information are not inconsistent with the elements required by this section.

(2) Defective authorizations. An authorization is not valid, if the document submitted has any of the following defects:

(i) The expiration date has passed or the expiration event is known by the covered entity to have occurred;

(ii) The authorization has not been filled out completely, with respect to an element described by paragraph (c) of this section, if applicable;

(iii) The authorization is known by the covered entity to have been revoked;

(iv) The authorization violates paragraph (b)(3) or (4) of this section, if applicable;

(v) Any material information in the authorization is known by the covered entity to be false.

(3) Compound authorizations. An authorization for use or disclosure of protected health information may not be combined with any other document to create a compound authorization, except as follows:

(i) An authorization for the use or disclosure of protected health information for a research study may be combined with any other type of written permission for the same research study, including another authorization for the use or disclosure of protected health information for such research or a consent to participate in such research;

(ii) An authorization for a use or disclosure of psychotherapy notes may only be combined with another authorization for a use or disclosure of psychotherapy notes;

(iii) An authorization under this section, other than an authorization for a use or disclosure of psychotherapy notes, may be combined with any other such authorization under this section, except when a covered entity has conditioned the provision of treatment, payment, enrollment in the health plan, or eligibility for benefits under paragraph (b)(4) of this section on the provision of one of the authorizations.

(4) Prohibition on conditioning of authorizations. A covered entity may not condition the provision to an individual of treatment, payment, enrollment in the health plan, or eligibility for benefits on the provision of an authorization, except:

(i) A covered health care provider may condition the provision of research-related treatment on provision of an authorization for the use or disclosure of protected health information for such research under this section;

(ii) A health plan may condition enrollment in the health plan or eligibility for benefits on provision of an authorization requested by the health plan prior to an individual's enrollment in the health plan, if:

(A) The authorization sought is for the health plan's eligibility or enrollment determinations relating to the individual or for its underwriting or risk rating determinations; and

(B) The authorization is not for a use or disclosure of psychotherapy notes under paragraph (a)(2) of this section; and

(iii) A covered entity may condition the provision of health care that is solely for the purpose of creating protected health information for disclosure to a third party on provision of an authorization for the disclosure of the protected health information to such third party.

(5) Revocation of authorizations. An individual may revoke an authorization provided under this section at any time, provided that the revocation is in writing, except to the extent that:

(i) The covered entity has taken action in reliance thereon; or

(ii) If the authorization was obtained as a condition of obtaining insurance coverage, other law provides the insurer with the right to contest a claim under the policy or the policy itself.

(6) Documentation. A covered entity must document and retain any signed authorization under this section as required by §164.530(j).

(c) Implementation specifications: Core elements and requirements.

(1) Core elements. A valid authorization under this section must contain at least the following elements:

(i) A description of the information to be used or disclosed that identifies the information in a specific and meaningful fashion.

(ii) The name or other specific identification of the person(s), or class of persons, authorized to make the requested use or disclosure.

(iii) The name or other specific identification of the person(s), or class of persons, to whom the covered entity may make the requested use or disclosure.

(iv) A description of each purpose of the requested use or disclosure. The statement "at the request of the individual" is a sufficient description of the purpose when an individual initiates the authorization and does not, or elects not to, provide a statement of the purpose.

(v) An expiration date or an expiration event that relates to the individual or the purpose of the use or disclosure. The statement "end of the research study," "none," or similar language is sufficient if the authorization is for a use or disclosure of protected health information for research, including for the creation and maintenance of a research database or research repository.

(vi) Signature of the individual and date. If the authorization is signed by a personal representative of the individual, a description of such representative's authority to act for the individual must also be provided.

(2) Required statements. In addition to the core elements, the authorization must contain statements adequate to place the individual on notice of all of the following:

(i) The individual's right to revoke the authorization in writing, and either:

(A) The exceptions to the right to revoke and a description of how the individual may revoke the authorization; or

(B) To the extent that the information in paragraph (c)(2)(i)(A) of this section is included in the notice required by §164.520, a reference to the covered entity's notice.

(ii) The ability or inability to condition treatment, payment, enrollment or eligibility for benefits on the authorization, by stating either:

(A) The covered entity may not condition treatment, payment, enrollment or eligibility for benefits on whether the individual signs the authorization when the prohibition on conditioning of authorizations in paragraph (b)(4) of this section applies; or

(B) The consequences to the individual of a refusal to sign the authorization when, in accordance with paragraph (b)(4) of this section, the covered entity can condition treatment, enrollment in the health plan, or eligibility for benefits on failure to obtain such authorization.

(iii) The potential for information disclosed pursuant to the authorization to be subject to redisclosure by the recipient and no longer be protected by this subpart.

(3) Plain language requirement. The authorization must be written in plain language.

(4) Copy to the individual. If a covered entity seeks an authorization from an individual for a use or disclosure of protected health information, the covered entity must provide the individual with a copy of the signed authorization.

§164.510 Uses and disclosures requiring an opportunity for the individual to agree or to object.

A covered entity may use or disclose protected health information, provided that the individual is informed in advance of the use or disclosure and has the opportunity to agree to or prohibit or restrict the use or disclosure, in accordance with the applicable requirements of this section. The covered entity may orally inform the individual of and obtain the individual's oral agreement or objection to a use or disclosure permitted by this section.

(a) Standard: use and disclosure for facility directories.

(1) Permitted uses and disclosure. Except when an objection is expressed in accordance with paragraphs (a)(2) or (3) of this section, a covered health care provider may:

(i) Use the following protected health information to maintain a directory of individuals in its facility:

(A) The individual's name;

(B) The individual's location in the covered health care provider's facility;

(C) The individual's condition described in general terms that does not communicate specific medical information about the individual; and

(D) The individual's religious affiliation; and

(ii) Disclose for directory purposes such information:

(A) To members of the clergy; or

(B) Except for religious affiliation, to other persons who ask for the individual by name.

(2) Opportunity to object. A covered health care provider must inform an individual of the protected health information that it may include in a directory and the persons to whom it may disclose such information (including disclosures to clergy of information regarding religious affiliation) and provide the individual with the opportunity to restrict or prohibit some or all of the uses or disclosures permitted by paragraph (a)(1) of this section.

(3) Emergency circumstances.

(i) If the opportunity to object to uses or disclosures required by paragraph (a)(2) of this section cannot practicably be provided because of the individual's incapacity or an emergency treatment circumstance, a covered health care provider may use or disclose some or all of the protected health information permitted by paragraph (a)(1) of this section for the facility's directory, if such disclosure is:

(A) Consistent with a prior expressed preference of the individual, if any, that is known to the covered health care provider; and

(B) In the individual's best interest as determined by the covered health care provider, in the exercise of professional judgment.

(ii) The covered health care provider must inform the individual and provide an opportunity to object to uses or disclosures for directory purposes as required by paragraph (a)(2) of this section when it becomes practicable to do so.

(b) Standard: uses and disclosures for involvement in the individual's care and notification purposes.

(1) Permitted uses and disclosures.

(i) A covered entity may, in accordance with paragraphs (b)(2) or (3) of this section, disclose to a family member, other relative, or a close personal friend of the individual, or any other person identified by the individual, the protected health information directly relevant to such person's involvement with the individual's care or payment related to the individual's health care.

(ii) A covered entity may use or disclose protected health information to notify, or assist in the notification of (including identifying or locating), a family member, a personal representative of the individual, or another person responsible for the care of the individual of the individual's location, general condition, or death. Any such use or disclosure of protected health information for such notification purposes must be in accordance with paragraphs (b)(2), (3), or (4) of this section, as applicable.

(2) Uses and disclosures with the individual present. If the individual is present for, or otherwise available prior to, a use or disclosure permitted by paragraph (b)(1) of this section and has the capacity to make health

care decisions, the covered entity may use or disclose the protected health information if it:

> (i) Obtains the individual's agreement;

> (ii) Provides the individual with the opportunity to object to the disclosure, and the individual does not express an objection; or

> (iii) Reasonably infers from the circumstances, based the exercise of professional judgment, that the individual does not object to the disclosure.

(3) Limited uses and disclosures when the individual is not present. If the individual is not present, or the opportunity to agree or object to the use or disclosure cannot practicably be provided because of the individual's incapacity or an emergency circumstance, the covered entity may, in the exercise of professional judgment, determine whether the disclosure is in the best interests of the individual and, if so, disclose only the protected health information that is directly relevant to the person's involvement with the individual's health care. A covered entity may use professional judgment and its experience with common practice to make reasonable inferences of the individual's best interest in allowing a person to act on behalf of the individual to pick up filled prescriptions, medical supplies, X-rays, or other similar forms of protected health information.

(4) Use and disclosures for disaster relief purposes. A covered entity may use or disclose protected health information to a public or private entity authorized by law or by its charter to assist in disaster relief efforts, for the purpose of coordinating with such entities the uses or disclosures permitted by paragraph (b)(1)(ii) of this section. The requirements in paragraphs (b)(2) and (3) of this section apply to such uses and disclosure to the extent that the covered entity, in the exercise of professional judgment, determines that the requirements do not interfere with the ability to respond to the emergency circumstances.

§164.512 Uses and disclosures for which an authorization or opportunity to agree or object is not required.

A covered entity may use or disclose protected health information without the written authorization of the individual, as described in §164.508, or the opportunity for the individual to agree or object as described in §164.510, in the situations covered by this section, subject to the applicable requirements of this section. When the covered entity is required by this section to inform the individual of, or when the individual may agree to, a use or disclosure permitted by this section, the covered entity's information and the individual's agreement may be given orally.

(a) Standard: uses and disclosures required by law.

(1) A covered entity may use or disclose protected health information to the extent that such use or disclosure is required by law and the use or disclosure complies with and is limited to the relevant requirements of such law.

(2) A covered entity must meet the requirements described in paragraph (c), (e), or (f) of this section for uses or disclosures required by law.

(b) Standard: uses and disclosures for public health activities.

(1) Permitted disclosures. A covered entity may disclose protected health information for the public health activities and purposes described in this paragraph to:

(i) A public health authority that is authorized by law to collect or receive such information for the purpose of preventing or controlling disease, injury, or disability, including, but not limited to, the reporting of disease, injury, vital events such as birth or death, and the conduct of public health surveillance, public health investigations, and public health interventions; or, at the direction of a public health authority, to an official of a foreign government agency that is acting in collaboration with a public health authority;

(ii) A public health authority or other appropriate government authority authorized by law to receive reports of child abuse or neglect;

(iii) A person subject to the jurisdiction of the Food and Drug Administration (FDA) with respect to an FDA-regulated product or activity for which that person has responsibility, for the purpose of activities related to the quality, safety or effectiveness of such FDA-regulated product or activity. Such purposes include:

(A) To collect or report adverse events (or similar activities with respect to food or dietary supplements), product defects or problems (including problems with the use or labeling of a product), or biological product deviations;

(B) To track FDA-regulated products;

(C) To enable product recalls, repairs, or replacement, or look-back (including locating and notifying individuals who have received products that have been recalled, withdrawn, or are the subject of lookback); or

(D) To conduct post marketing surveillance;

(iv) A person who may have been exposed to a communicable disease or may otherwise be at risk of contracting or spreading a disease or condition, if the covered entity or public health authority is authorized by law to notify such person as necessary in the conduct of a public health intervention or investigation; or

(v) An employer, about an individual who is a member of the workforce of the employer, if:

(A) The covered entity is a covered health care provider who is a member of the workforce of such employer or who provides health care to the individual at the request of the employer:

(1) To conduct an evaluation relating to medical surveillance of the workplace; or

(2) To evaluate whether the individual has a work-related illness or injury;

(B) The protected health information that is disclosed consists of findings concerning a work-related illness or injury or a workplace-related medical surveillance;

(C) The employer needs such findings in order to comply with its obligations, under 29 CFR parts 1904 through 1928, 30 CFR parts 50 through 90, or under state law having a similar purpose, to record such illness or injury or to carry out responsibilities for workplace medical surveillance; and

(D) The covered health care provider provides written notice to the individual that protected health information relating to the medical surveillance of the workplace and work-related illnesses and injuries is disclosed to the employer:

(1) By giving a copy of the notice to the individual at the time the health care is provided; or

(2) If the health care is provided on the work site of the employer, by posting the notice in a prominent place at the location where the health care is provided.

(2) Permitted uses. If the covered entity also is a public health authority, the covered entity is permitted to use protected health information in all cases in which it is permitted to disclose such information for public health activities under paragraph (b)(1) of this section.

(c) Standard: disclosures about victims of abuse, neglect or domestic violence.

(1) Permitted disclosures. Except for reports of child abuse or neglect permitted by paragraph (b)(1)(ii) of this section, a covered entity may disclose protected health information about an individual whom the covered entity reasonably believes to be a victim of abuse, neglect, or domestic violence to a government authority, including a social service or protective services agency, authorized by law to receive reports of such abuse, neglect, or domestic violence:

(i) To the extent the disclosure is required by law and the disclosure complies with and is limited to the relevant requirements of such law;

(ii) If the individual agrees to the disclosure; or

(iii) To the extent the disclosure is expressly authorized by statute or regulation and:

(A) The covered entity, in the exercise of professional judgment, believes the disclosure is necessary to prevent serious harm to the individual or other potential victims; or

(B) If the individual is unable to agree because of incapacity, a law enforcement or other public official authorized to receive the report represents that the protected health information for which disclosure is sought is not intended to be used against the individual and that an immediate enforcement activity that depends upon the disclosure would be materially and adversely affected by waiting until the individual is able to agree to the disclosure.

(2) Informing the individual. A covered entity that makes a disclosure permitted by paragraph (c)(1) of this section must promptly inform the individual that such a report has been or will be made, except if:

(i) The covered entity, in the exercise of professional judgment, believes informing the individual would place the individual at risk of serious harm; or

(ii) The covered entity would be informing a personal representative, and the covered entity reasonably believes the personal representative is responsible for the abuse, neglect, or other injury, and that informing such person would not be in the best interests of the individual as determined by the covered entity, in the exercise of professional judgment.

(d) Standard: uses and disclosures for health oversight activities.

(1) Permitted disclosures. A covered entity may disclose protected health information to a health oversight agency for oversight activities authorized by law, including audits; civil, administrative, or criminal investigations; inspections; licensure or disciplinary actions; civil, administrative, or criminal proceedings or actions; or other activities necessary for appropriate oversight of:

(i) The health care system;

(ii) Government benefit programs for which health information is relevant to beneficiary eligibility;

(iii) Entities subject to government regulatory programs for which health information is necessary for determining compliance with program standards; or

(iv) Entities subject to civil rights laws for which health information is necessary for determining compliance.

(2) Exception to health oversight activities. For the purpose of the disclosures permitted by paragraph (d)(1) of this section, a health oversight activity does not include an investigation or other activity in which the individual is the subject of the investigation or activity and such investigation or other activity does not arise out of and is not directly related to:

(i) The receipt of health care;

(ii) A claim for public benefits related to health; or

(iii) Qualification for, or receipt of, public benefits or services when a patient's health is integral to the claim for public benefits or services.

(3) Joint activities or investigations. Nothwithstanding paragraph (d)(2) of this section, if a health oversight activity or investigation is conducted in conjunction with an oversight activity or investigation relating to a claim for public benefits not related to health, the joint activity or investigation is considered a health oversight activity for purposes of paragraph (d) of this section.

(4) Permitted uses. If a covered entity also is a health oversight agency, the covered entity may use protected health information for health oversight activities as permitted by paragraph (d) of this section.

(e) Standard: disclosures for judicial and administrative proceedings.

(1) Permitted disclosures. A covered entity may disclose protected health information in the course of any judicial or administrative proceeding:

(i) In response to an order of a court or administrative tribunal, provided that the covered entity discloses only the protected health information expressly authorized by such order; or

(ii) In response to a subpoena, discovery request, or other lawful process, that is not accompanied by an order of a court or administrative tribunal, if:

(A) The covered entity receives satisfactory assurance, as described in paragraph (e)(1)(iii) of this section, from the party seeking the information that reasonable efforts have been made by such party to ensure that the individual who is the subject of the protected health information that has been requested has been given notice of the request; or

(B) The covered entity receives satisfactory assurance, as described in paragraph (e)(1)(iv) of this section, from the party seeking the information that reasonable efforts have been made by such party to secure a qualified protective order that meets the requirements of paragraph (e)(1)(v) of this section.

(iii) For the purposes of paragraph (e)(1)(ii)(A) of this section, a covered entity receives satisfactory assurances from a party seeking protecting health information if the covered entity receives from such party a written statement and accompanying documentation demonstrating that:

(A) The party requesting such information has made a good faith attempt to provide written notice to the individual (or, if the individual's location is unknown, to mail a notice to the individual's last known address);

(B) The notice included sufficient information about the litigation or proceeding in which the protected health information is requested to permit the individual to raise an objection to the court or administrative tribunal; and

(C) The time for the individual to raise objections to the court or administrative tribunal has elapsed, and:

(1) No objections were filed; or

(2) All objections filed by the individual have been resolved by the court or the administrative tribunal and the disclosures being sought are consistent with such resolution.

(iv) For the purposes of paragraph (e)(1)(ii)(B) of this section, a covered entity receives satisfactory assurances from a party seeking protected health information, if the covered entity receives from such party a written statement and accompanying documentation demonstrating that:

(A) The parties to the dispute giving rise to the request for information have agreed to a qualified protective order and have presented it to the court or administrative tribunal with jurisdiction over the dispute; or

(B) The party seeking the protected health information has requested a qualified protective order from such court or administrative tribunal.

(v) For purposes of paragraph (e)(1) of this section, a qualified protective order means, with respect to protected health information requested under paragraph (e)(1)(ii) of this section, an order of a court or of an administrative tribunal or a stipulation by the parties to the litigation or administrative proceeding that:

(A) Prohibits the parties from using or disclosing the protected health information for any purpose other than the litigation or proceeding for which such information was requested; and

(B) Requires the return to the covered entity or destruction of the protected health information (including all copies made) at the end of the litigation or proceeding.

(vi) Notwithstanding paragraph (e)(1)(ii) of this section, a covered entity may disclose protected health information in response to lawful process described in paragraph (e)(1)(ii) of this section without receiving satisfactory assurance under paragraph (e)(1)(ii)(A) or (B) of this section, if the covered entity makes reasonable efforts to provide notice to the individual sufficient to meet the requirements of paragraph (e)(1)(iii) of this section or to seek a qualified protective order sufficient to meet the requirements of paragraph (e)(1)(iv) of this section.

(2) Other uses and disclosures under this section. The provisions of this paragraph do not supersede other provisions of this section that otherwise permit or restrict uses or disclosures of protected health information.

(f) Standard: disclosures for law enforcement purposes. A covered entity may disclose protected health information for a law enforcement purpose to a law enforcement official if the conditions in paragraphs (f)(1) through (f)(6) of this section are met, as applicable.

(1) Permitted disclosures: pursuant to process and as otherwise required by law. A covered entity may disclose protected health information:

(i) As required by law including laws that require the reporting of certain types of wounds or other physical injuries, except for laws subject to paragraph (b)(1)(ii) or (c)(1)(i) of this section; or

(ii) In compliance with and as limited by the relevant requirements of:

(A) A court order or court-ordered warrant, or a subpoena or summons issued by a judicial officer;

(B) A grand jury subpoena; or

(C) An administrative request, including an administrative subpoena or summons, a civil or an authorized investigative demand, or similar process authorized under law, provided that:

(1) The information sought is relevant and material to a legitimate law enforcement inquiry;

(2) The request is specific and limited in scope to the extent reasonably practicable in light of the purpose for which the information is sought; and

(3) De-identified information could not reasonably be used.

(2) Permitted disclosures: limited information for identification and location purposes. Except for disclosures required by law as permitted by paragraph (f)(1) of this section, a covered entity may disclose protected health information in response to a law enforcement official's request for such information for the purpose of identifying or locating a suspect, fugitive, material witness, or missing person, provided that:

(i) The covered entity may disclose only the following information:

(A) Name and address;

(B) Date and place of birth;

(C) Social security number;

(D) ABO blood type and rh factor;

(E) Type of injury;

(F) Date and time of treatment;

(G) Date and time of death, if applicable; and

(H) A description of distinguishing physical characteristics, including height, weight, gender, race, hair and eye color, presence or absence of facial hair (beard or moustache), scars, and tattoos.

(ii) Except as permitted by paragraph (f)(2)(i) of this section, the covered entity may not disclose for the purposes of identification or location under paragraph (f)(2) of this section any protected health information related to the individual's DNA or DNA analysis, dental records, or typing, samples or analysis of body fluids or tissue.

(3) Permitted disclosure: victims of a crime. Except for disclosures required by law as permitted by paragraph (f)(1) of this section, a covered entity may disclose protected health information in response to a law enforcement official's request for such information about an individual who is or is suspected to be a victim of a crime, other than disclosures that are subject to paragraph (b) or (c) of this section, if:

(i) The individual agrees to the disclosure; or

(ii) The covered entity is unable to obtain the individual's agreement because of incapacity or other emergency circumstance, provided that:

(A) The law enforcement official represents that such information is needed to determine whether a violation of law by a person other than the victim has occurred, and such information is not intended to be used against the victim;

(B) The law enforcement official represents that immediate law enforcement activity that depends upon the disclosure would be materially and adversely affected by waiting until the individual is able to agree to the disclosure; and

(C) The disclosure is in the best interests of the individual as determined by the covered entity, in the exercise of professional judgment.

(4) Permitted disclosure: decedents. A covered entity may disclose protected health information about an individual who has died to a law enforcement official for the purpose of alerting law enforcement of the death of the individual if the covered entity has a suspicion that such death may have resulted from criminal conduct.

(5) Permitted disclosure: crime on premises. A covered entity may disclose to a law enforcement official protected health information that the covered entity believes in good faith constitutes evidence of criminal conduct that occurred on the premises of the covered entity.

(6) Permitted disclosure: reporting crime in emergencies.

(i) A covered health care provider providing emergency health care in response to a medical emergency, other than such emergency on the premises of the covered health care provider, may disclose protected health information to a law enforcement official if such disclosure appears necessary to alert law enforcement to:

(A) The commission and nature of a crime;

(B) The location of such crime or of the victim(s) of such crime; and

(C) The identity, description, and location of the perpetrator of such crime.

(ii) If a covered health care provider believes that the medical emergency described in paragraph (f)(6)(i) of this section is the result of abuse, neglect, or domestic violence of the individual in need of emergency health care, paragraph (f)(6)(i) of this section does not apply and any disclosure to a law enforcement official for law enforcement purposes is subject to paragraph (c) of this section.

(g) Standard: uses and disclosures about decedents.

(1) Coroners and medical examiners. A covered entity may disclose protected health information to a coroner or medical examiner for the purpose of identifying a deceased person, determining a cause of death, or other duties as authorized by law. A covered entity that also performs the duties of a coroner or medical examiner may use protected health information for the purposes described in this paragraph.

(2) Funeral directors. A covered entity may disclose protected health information to funeral directors, consistent with applicable law, as necessary to carry out their duties with respect to the decedent. If necessary for funeral directors to carry out their duties, the covered entity may disclose the protected health information prior to, and in reasonable anticipation of, the individual's death.

(h) Standard: uses and disclosures for cadaveric organ, eye or tissue donation purposes. A covered entity may use or disclose protected health information to organ procurement organizations or other entities engaged in the procurement, banking, or transplantation of cadaveric organs, eyes, or tissue for the purpose of facilitating organ, eye or tissue donation and transplantation.

(i) Standard: uses and disclosures for research purposes.

(1) Permitted uses and disclosures. A covered entity may use or disclose protected health information for research, regardless of the source of funding of the research, provided that:

(i) Board approval of a waiver of authorization. The covered entity obtains documentation that an alteration to or waiver, in whole or in part, of the individual authorization required by §164.508 for use or disclosure of protected health information has been approved by either:

(A) An Institutional Review Board (IRB), established in accordance with 7 CFR 1c.107, 10 CFR 745.107, 14 CFR 1230.107, 15 CFR 27.107, 16 CFR 1028.107, 21 CFR 56.107, 22 CFR 225.107, 24 CFR 60.107, 28 CFR 46.107, 32 CFR 219.107, 34 CFR 97.107,

38 CFR 16.107, 40 CFR 26.107, 45 CFR 46.107, 45 CFR 690.107, or 49 CFR 11.107; or

(B) A privacy board that:

(1) Has members with varying backgrounds and appropriate professional competency as necessary to review the effect of the research protocol on the individual's privacy rights and related interests;

(2) Includes at least one member who is not affiliated with the covered entity, not affiliated with any entity conducting or sponsoring the research, and not related to any person who is affiliated with any of such entities; and

(3) Does not have any member participating in a review of any project in which the member has a conflict of interest.

(ii) Reviews preparatory to research. The covered entity obtains from the researcher representations that:

(A) Use or disclosure is sought solely to review protected health information as necessary to prepare a research protocol or for similar purposes preparatory to research;

(B) No protected health information is to be removed from the covered entity by the researcher in the course of the review; and

(C) The protected health information for which use or access is sought is necessary for the research purposes.

(iii) Research on decedent's information. The covered entity obtains from the researcher:

(A) Representation that the use or disclosure sought is solely for research on the protected health information of decedents;

(B) Documentation, at the request of the covered entity, of the death of such individuals; and

(C) Representation that the protected health information for which use or disclosure is sought is necessary for the research purposes.

(2) Documentation of waiver approval. For a use or disclosure to be permitted based on documentation of approval of an alteration or waiver,

under paragraph (i)(1)(i) of this section, the documentation must include all of the following:

(i) Identification and date of action. A statement identifying the IRB or privacy board and the date on which the alteration or waiver of authorization was approved;

(ii) Waiver criteria. A statement that the IRB or privacy board has determined that the alteration or waiver, in whole or in part, of authorization satisfies the following criteria:

(A) The use or disclosure of protected health information involves no more than a minimal risk to the privacy of individuals, based on, at least, the presence of the following elements;

(1) An adequate plan to protect the identifiers from improper use and disclosure;

(2) An adequate plan to destroy the identifiers at the earliest opportunity consistent with conduct of the research, unless there is a health or research justification for retaining the identifiers or such retention is otherwise required by law; and

(3) Adequate written assurances that the protected health information will not be reused or disclosed to any other person or entity, except as required by law, for authorized oversight of the research study, or for other research for which the use or disclosure of protected health information would be permitted by this subpart;

(B) The research could not practicably be conducted without the waiver or alteration; and

(C) The research could not practicably be conducted without access to and use of the protected health information.

(iii) Protected health information needed. A brief description of the protected health information for which use or access has been determined to be necessary by the IRB or privacy board has determined, pursuant to paragraph (i)(2)(ii)(C) of this section;

(iv) Review and approval procedures. A statement that the alteration or waiver of authorization has been reviewed and approved under either normal or expedited review procedures, as follows:

(A) An IRB must follow the requirements of the Common Rule, including the normal review procedures (7 CFR 1c.108(b), 10 CFR 745.108(b), 14 CFR 1230.108(b), 15 CFR 27.108(b), 16 1028.108(b), 21 CFR 56.108(b), 22 CFR 225.108(b), 24 CFR 60.108(b), 28 CFR 46.108(b), 32 CFR 219.108(b), 34 CFR 97.108(b), 38 CFR 16.108(b), 40 CFR 26.108(b), 45 CFR 46.108(b), 45 CFR 690.108(b), or 49 CFR 11.108(b)) or the expedited review procedures (7 CFR 1c.110, 10 CFR 745.110, 14 CFR 1230.110, 15 CFR 27.110, 16 CFR 1028.110, 21 CFR 56.110, 22 CFR 225.110, 24 CFR 60.110, 28 CFR 46.110, 32 CFR 219.110, 34 CFR 97.110, 38 CFR 16.110, 40 CFR 26.110, 45 CFR 46.110, 45 CFR 690.110, or 49 CFR 11.110);

(B) A privacy board must review the proposed research at convened meetings at which a majority of the privacy board members are present, including at least one member who satisfies the criterion stated in paragraph (i)(1)(i)(B)(2) of this section, and the alteration or waiver of authorization must be approved by the majority of the privacy board members present at the meeting, unless the privacy board elects to use an expedited review procedure in accordance with paragraph (i)(2)(iv)(C) of this section;

(C) A privacy board may use an expedited review procedure if the research involves no more than minimal risk to the privacy of the individuals who are the subject of the protected health information for which use or disclosure is being sought. If the privacy board elects to use an expedited review procedure, the review and approval of the alteration or waiver of authorization may be carried out by the chair of the privacy board, or by one or more members of the privacy board as designated by the chair; and

(v) Required signature. The documentation of the alteration or waiver of authorization must be signed by the chair or other member, as designated by the chair, of the IRB or the privacy board, as applicable.

(j) Standard: uses and disclosures to avert a serious threat to health or safety.

(1) Permitted disclosures. A covered entity may, consistent with applicable law and standards of ethical conduct, use or disclose protected health information, if the covered entity, in good faith, believes the use or disclosure:

(i)(A) Is necessary to prevent or lessen a serious and imminent threat to the health or safety of a person or the public; and

(B) Is to a person or persons reasonably able to prevent or lessen the threat, including the target of the threat; or

(ii) Is necessary for law enforcement authorities to identify or apprehend an individual:

(A) Because of a statement by an individual admitting participation in a violent crime that the covered entity reasonably believes may have caused serious physical harm to the victim; or

(B) Where it appears from all the circumstances that the individual has escaped from a correctional institution or from lawful custody, as those terms are defined in §164.501.

(2) Use or disclosure not permitted. A use or disclosure pursuant to paragraph (j)(1)(ii)(A) of this section may not be made if the information described in paragraph (j)(1)(ii)(A) of this section is learned by the covered entity:

(i) In the course of treatment to affect the propensity to commit the criminal conduct that is the basis for the disclosure under paragraph (j)(1)(ii)(A) of this section, or counseling or therapy; or

(ii) Through a request by the individual to initiate or to be referred for the treatment, counseling, or therapy described in paragraph (j)(2)(i) of this section.

(3) Limit on information that may be disclosed. A disclosure made pursuant to paragraph (j)(1)(ii)(A) of this section shall contain only the statement described in paragraph (j)(1)(ii)(A) of this section and the protected health information described in paragraph (f)(2)(i) of this section.

(4) Presumption of good faith belief. A covered entity that uses or discloses protected health information pursuant to paragraph (j)(1) of this section is presumed to have acted in good faith with regard to a belief described in paragraph (j)(1)(i) or (ii) of this section, if the belief is based upon the covered entity's actual knowledge or in reliance on a credible representation by a person with apparent knowledge or authority.

(k) Standard: uses and disclosures for specialized government functions.

(1) Military and veterans activities.

(i) Armed Forces personnel. A covered entity may use and disclose the protected health information of individuals who are Armed Forces personnel for activities deemed necessary by appropriate military command authorities to assure the proper execution of the military mission, if the appropriate military authority has published by notice in the Federal Register the following information:

(A) Appropriate military command authorities; and

(B) The purposes for which the protected health information may be used or disclosed.

(ii) Separation or discharge from military service. A covered entity that is a component of the Departments of Defense or Transportation may disclose to the Department of Veterans Affairs (DVA) the protected health information of an individual who is a member of the Armed Forces upon the separation or discharge of the individual from military service for the purpose of a determination by DVA of the individual's eligibility for or entitlement to benefits under laws administered by the Secretary of Veterans Affairs.

(iii) Veterans. A covered entity that is a component of the Department of Veterans Affairs may use and disclose protected health information to components of the Department that determine eligibility for or entitlement to, or that provide, benefits under the laws administered by the Secretary of Veterans Affairs.

(iv) Foreign military personnel. A covered entity may use and disclose the protected health information of individuals who are foreign military personnel to their appropriate foreign military authority for the same purposes for which uses and disclosures are permitted for Armed Forces personnel under the notice published in the Federal Register pursuant to paragraph (k)(1)(i) of this section.

(2) National security and intelligence activities. A covered entity may disclose protected health information to authorized federal officials for the conduct of lawful intelligence, counter-intelligence, and other national security activities authorized by the National Security Act (50 U.S.C. 401, et seq.) and implementing authority (e.g., Executive Order 12333).

(3) Protective services for the President and others. A covered entity may disclose protected health information to authorized federal officials for the provision of protective services to the President or other persons

authorized by 18 U.S.C. 3056, or to foreign heads of state or other persons authorized by 22 U.S.C. 2709(a)(3), or to for the conduct of investigations authorized by 18 U.S.C. 871 and 879.

(4) Medical suitability determinations. A covered entity that is a component of the Department of State may use protected health information to make medical suitability determinations and may disclose whether or not the individual was determined to be medically suitable to the officials in the Department of State who need access to such information for the following purposes:

(i) For the purpose of a required security clearance conducted pursuant to Executive Orders 10450 and 12698;

(ii) As necessary to determine worldwide availability or availability for mandatory service abroad under sections 101(a)(4) and 504 of the Foreign Service Act; or

(iii) For a family to accompany a Foreign Service member abroad, consistent with section 101(b)(5) and 904 of the Foreign Service Act.

(5) Correctional institutions and other law enforcement custodial situations.

(i) Permitted disclosures. A covered entity may disclose to a correctional institution or a law enforcement official having lawful custody of an inmate or other individual protected health information about such inmate or individual, if the correctional institution or such law enforcement official represents that such protected health information is necessary for:

(A) The provision of health care to such individuals;

(B) The health and safety of such individual or other inmates;

(C) The health and safety of the officers or employees of or others at the correctional institution;

(D) The health and safety of such individuals and officers or other persons responsible for the transporting of inmates or their transfer from one institution, facility, or setting to another;

(E) Law enforcement on the premises of the correctional institution; and

(F) The administration and maintenance of the safety, security, and good order of the correctional institution.

(ii) Permitted uses. A covered entity that is a correctional institution may use protected health information of individuals who are inmates for any purpose for which such protected health information may be disclosed.

(iii) No application after release. For the purposes of this provision, an individual is no longer an inmate when released on parole, probation, supervised release, or otherwise is no longer in lawful custody.

(6) Covered entities that are government programs providing public benefits.

(i) A health plan that is a government program providing public benefits may disclose protected health information relating to eligibility for or enrollment in the health plan to another agency administering a government program providing public benefits if the sharing of eligibility or enrollment information among such government agencies or the maintenance of such information in a single or combined data system accessible to all such government agencies is required or expressly authorized by statute or regulation.

(ii) A covered entity that is a government agency administering a government program providing public benefits may disclose protected health information relating to the program to another covered entity that is a government agency administering a government program providing public benefits if the programs serve the same or similar populations and the disclosure of protected health information is necessary to coordinate the covered functions of such programs or to improve administration and management relating to the covered functions of such programs.

(l) Standard: disclosures for workers' compensation. A covered entity may disclose protected health information as authorized by and to the extent necessary to comply with laws relating to workers' compensation or other similar programs, established by law, that provide benefits for work-related injuries or illness without regard to fault.

§164.514 Other requirements relating to uses and disclosures of protected health information.

(a) Standard: de-identification of protected health information. Health information that does not identify an individual and with respect to which there is no reasonable basis to believe that the information can be used to identify an individual is not individually identifiable health information.

(b) Implementation specifications: requirements for de-identification of protected health information. A covered entity may determine that health information is not individually identifiable health information only if:

(1) A person with appropriate knowledge of and experience with generally accepted statistical and scientific principles and methods for rendering information not individually identifiable:

(i) Applying such principles and methods, determines that the risk is very small that the information could be used, alone or in combination with other reasonably available information, by an anticipated recipient to identify an individual who is a subject of the information; and

(ii) Documents the methods and results of the analysis that justify such determination; or

(2)(i) The following identifiers of the individual or of relatives, employers, or household members of the individual, are removed:

(A) Names;

(B) All geographic subdivisions smaller than a State, including street address, city, county, precinct, zip code, and their equivalent geocodes, except for the initial three digits of a zip code if, according to the current publicly available data from the Bureau of the Census:

(1) The geographic unit formed by combining all zip codes with the same three initial digits contains more than 20,000 people; and

(2) The initial three digits of a zip code for all such geographic units containing 20,000 or fewer people is changed to 000.

(C) All elements of dates (except year) for dates directly related to an individual, including birth date, admission date, discharge date, date of death; and all ages over 89 and all elements of dates (including year) indicative of such age, except that such ages and elements may be aggregated into a single category of age 90 or older;

(D) Telephone numbers;

(E) Fax numbers;

(F) Electronic mail addresses;

(G) Social security numbers;

(H) Medical record numbers;

(I) Health plan beneficiary numbers;

(J) Account numbers;

(K) Certificate/license numbers;

(L) Vehicle identifiers and serial numbers, including license plate numbers;

(M) Device identifiers and serial numbers;

(N) Web Universal Resource Locators (URLs);

(O) Internet Protocol (IP) address numbers;

(P) Biometric identifiers, including finger and voice prints;

(Q) Full face photographic images and any comparable images; and

(R) Any other unique identifying number, characteristic, or code, except as permitted by paragraph (c) of this section; and

(ii) The covered entity does not have actual knowledge that the information could be used alone or in combination with other information to identify an individual who is a subject of the information.

(c) Implementation specifications: re-identification. A covered entity may assign a code or other means of record identification to allow information de-identified under this section to be re-identified by the covered entity, provided that:

(1) Derivation. The code or other means of record identification is not derived from or related to information about the individual and is not otherwise capable of being translated so as to identify the individual; and

(2) Security. The covered entity does not use or disclose the code or other means of record identification for any other purpose, and does not disclose the mechanism for re-identification.

(d)(1) Standard: minimum necessary requirements. In order to comply with §164.502(b) and this section, a covered entity must meet the requirements of paragraphs (d)(2) through (d)(5) of this section with respect to a request for, or the use and disclosure of, protected health information.

(2) Implementation specifications: minimum necessary uses of protected health information.

(i) A covered entity must identify:

(A) Those persons or classes of persons, as appropriate, in its workforce who need access to protected health information to carry out their duties; and

(B) For each such person or class of persons, the category or categories of protected health information to which access is needed and any conditions appropriate to such access.

(ii) A covered entity must make reasonable efforts to limit the access of such persons or classes identified in paragraph (d)(2)(i)(A) of this section to protected health information consistent with paragraph (d)(2)(i)(B) of this section.

(3) Implementation specification: minimum necessary disclosures of protected health information.

(i) For any type of disclosure that it makes on a routine and recurring basis, a covered entity must implement policies and procedures (which may be standard protocols) that limit the protected health information disclosed to the amount reasonably necessary to achieve the purpose of the disclosure.

(ii) For all other disclosures, a covered entity must:

(A) Develop criteria designed to limit the protected health information disclosed to the information reasonably necessary to accomplish the purpose for which disclosure is sought; and

(B) Review requests for disclosure on an individual basis in accordance with such criteria.

(iii) A covered entity may rely, if such reliance is reasonable under the circumstances, on a requested disclosure as the minimum necessary for the stated purpose when:

(A) Making disclosures to public officials that are permitted under §164.512, if the public official represents that the information requested is the minimum necessary for the stated purpose(s);

(B) The information is requested by another covered entity;

(C) The information is requested by a professional who is a member of its workforce or is a business associate of the covered entity for the purpose of providing professional services to the covered entity, if the professional represents that the information requested is the minimum necessary for the stated purpose(s); or

(D) Documentation or representations that comply with the applicable requirements of §164.512(i) have been provided by a person requesting the information for research purposes.

(4) Implementation specifications: minimum necessary requests for protected health information.

(i) A covered entity must limit any request for protected health information to that which is reasonably necessary to accomplish the purpose for which the request is made, when requesting such information from other covered entities.

(ii) For a request that is made on a routine and recurring basis, a covered entity must implement policies and procedures (which may be standard protocols) that limit the protected health information requested to the amount reasonably necessary to accomplish the purpose for which the request is made.

(iii) For all other requests, a covered entity must:

(A) Develop criteria designed to limit the request for protected health information to the information reasonably necessary to accomplish the purpose for which the request is made; and

(B) Review requests for disclosure on an individual basis in accordance with such criteria.

(5) Implementation specification: other content requirement. For all uses, disclosures, or requests to which the requirements in paragraph (d) of this section apply, a covered entity may not use, disclose or request an entire medical record, except when the entire medical record is specifically justified as the amount that is reasonably necessary to accomplish the purpose of the use, disclosure, or request.

(e) (1) Standard: Limited data set. A covered entity may use or disclose a limited data set that meets the requirements of paragraphs (e)(2) and (e)(3) of this section, if the covered entity enters into a data use agreement with the limited data set recipient, in accordance with paragraph (e)(4) of this section.

(2) Implementation specification: Limited data set: A limited data set is protected health information that excludes the following direct identifiers of the individual or of relatives, employers, or household members of the individual:

(i) Names;

(ii) Postal address information, other than town or city, State, and zip code;

(iii) Telephone numbers;

(iv) Fax numbers;

(v) Electronic mail addresses;

(vi) Social security numbers;

(vii) Medical record numbers;

(viii) Health plan beneficiary numbers;

(ix) Account numbers;

(x) Certificate/license numbers;

(xi) Vehicle identifiers and serial numbers, including license plate numbers;

(xii) Device identifiers and serial numbers;

(xiii) Web Universal Resource Locators (URLs);

(xiv) Internet Protocol (IP) address numbers;

(xv) Biometric identifiers, including finger and voice prints; and

(xvi) Full face photographic images and any comparable images.

(3) Implementation specification: Permitted purposes for uses and disclosures.

(i) A covered entity may use or disclose a limited data set under paragraph (e)(1) of this section only for the purposes of research, public health, or health care operations.

(ii) A covered entity may use protected health information to create a limited data set that meets the requirements of paragraph (e)(2) of this section, or disclose protected health information only to a business associate for such purpose, whether or not the limited data set is to be used by the covered entity.

(4) Implementation specifications: Data use agreement.

(i) Agreement required. A covered entity may use or disclose a limited data set under paragraph (e)(1) of this section only if the covered entity obtains satisfactory assurance, in the form of a data use agreement that meets the requirements of this section, that the limited data set recipient will only use or disclose the protected health information for limited purposes.

(ii) Contents. A data use agreement between the covered entity and the limited data set recipient must:

(A) Establish the permitted uses and disclosures of such information by the limited data set recipient, consistent with paragraph (e)(3) of this section. The data use agreement may not authorize the limited data set recipient to use or further disclose the information in a manner that would violate the requirements of this subpart, if done by the covered entity;

(B) Establish who is permitted to use or receive the limited data set; and

(C) Provide that the limited data set recipient will:

(1) Not use or further disclose the information other than as permitted by the data use agreement or as otherwise required by law;

(2) Use appropriate safeguards to prevent use or disclosure of the information other than as provided for by the data use agreement;

(3) Report to the covered entity any use or disclosure of the information not provided for by its data use agreement of which it becomes aware;

(4) Ensure that any agents, including a subcontractor, to whom it provides the limited data set agrees to the same restrictions and conditions that apply to the limited data set recipient with respect to such information; and

(5) Not identify the information or contact the individuals.

(iii) Compliance.

(A) A covered entity is not in compliance with the standards in paragraph (e) of this section if the covered entity knew of a pattern of activity or practice of the limited data set recipient that constituted a material breach or violation of the data use agreement, unless the covered entity took reasonable steps to cure the breach or end the violation, as applicable, and, if such steps were unsuccessful:

(1) Discontinued disclosure of protected health information to the recipient; and

(2) Reported the problem to the Secretary.

(B) A covered entity that is a limited data set recipient and violates a data use agreement will be in noncompliance with the standards, implementation specifications, and requirements of paragraph (e) of this section.

(f)(1) Standard: uses and disclosures for fundraising. A covered entity may use, or disclose to a business associate or to an institutionally related foundation, the following protected health information for the purpose of raising funds for its own benefit, without an authorization meeting the requirements of §164.508:

(i) Demographic information relating to an individual; and

(ii) Dates of health care provided to an individual.

(2) Implementation specifications: fundraising requirements.

(i) The covered entity may not use or disclose protected health information for fundraising purposes as otherwise permitted by paragraph (f)(1) of this section unless a statement required by §164.520(b)(1)(iii)(B) is included in the covered entity's notice;

(ii) The covered entity must include in any fundraising materials it sends to an individual under this paragraph a description of how the individual may opt out of receiving any further fundraising communications.

(iii) The covered entity must make reasonable efforts to ensure that individuals who decide to opt out of receiving future fundraising communications are not sent such communications.

(g) Standard: uses and disclosures for underwriting and related purposes. If a health plan receives protected heath information for the purpose of underwriting, premium rating, or other activities relating to the creation, renewal, or replacement of a contract of health insurance or health benefits, and if such health insurance or health benefits are not placed with the health plan, such health plan may not use or disclose such protected health information for any other purpose, except as may be required by law.

(h)(1) Standard: verification requirements. Prior to any disclosure permitted by this subpart, a covered entity must:

(i) Except with respect to disclosures under §164.510, verify the identity of a person requesting protected health information and the authority of any such person to have access to protected health information under this subpart, if the identity or any such authority of such person is not known to the covered entity; and

(ii) Obtain any documentation, statements, or representations, whether oral or written, from the person requesting the protected health information when such documentation, statement, or representation is a condition of the disclosure under this subpart.

(2) Implementation specifications: verification.

(i) Conditions on disclosures. If a disclosure is conditioned by this subpart on particular documentation, statements, or representations from the person requesting the protected health information, a covered entity may rely, if such reliance is reasonable under the circumstances, on documentation, statements, or representations that, on their face, meet the applicable requirements.

(A) The conditions in §164.512(f)(1)(ii)(C) may be satisfied by the administrative subpoena or similar process or by a separate written statement that, on its face, demonstrates that the applicable requirements have been met.

(B) The documentation required by §164.512(i)(2) may be satisfied by one or more written statements, provided that each is appropriately dated and signed in accordance with §164.512(i)(2)(i) and (v).

(ii) Identity of public officials. A covered entity may rely, if such reliance is reasonable under the circumstances, on any of the following to verify identity when the disclosure of protected health information is to a public official or a person acting on behalf of the public official:

(A) If the request is made in person, presentation of an agency identification badge, other official credentials, or other proof of government status;

(B) If the request is in writing, the request is on the appropriate government letterhead; or

(C) If the disclosure is to a person acting on behalf of a public official, a written statement on appropriate government letterhead that the person is acting under the government's authority or other evidence or documentation of agency, such as a contract for services, memorandum of understanding, or purchase order, that establishes that the person is acting on behalf of the public official.

(iii) Authority of public officials. A covered entity may rely, if such reliance is reasonable under the circumstances, on any of the following to verify authority when the disclosure of protected health information is to a public official or a person acting on behalf of the public official:

(A) A written statement of the legal authority under which the information is requested, or, if a written statement would be impracticable, an oral statement of such legal authority;

(B) If a request is made pursuant to legal process, warrant, subpoena, order, or other legal process issued by a grand jury or a judicial or administrative tribunal is presumed to constitute legal authority.

(iv) Exercise of professional judgment. The verification requirements of this paragraph are met if the covered entity relies on the exercise of professional judgment in making a use or disclosure in accordance with §164.510 or acts on a good faith belief in making a disclosure in accordance with §164.512(j).

§164.520 Notice of privacy practices for protected health information.

(a) Standard: notice of privacy practices.

(1) Right to notice. Except as provided by paragraph (a)(2) or (3) of this section, an individual has a right to adequate notice of the uses and disclosures of protected health information that may be made by the covered entity, and of the individual's rights and the covered entity's legal duties with respect to protected health information.

(2) Exception for group health plans.

(i) An individual enrolled in a group health plan has a right to notice:

(A) From the group health plan, if, and to the extent that, such an individual does not receive health benefits under the group health plan through an insurance contract with a health insurance issuer or HMO; or

(B) From the health insurance issuer or HMO with respect to the group health plan though which such individuals receive their health benefits under the group health plan.

(ii) A group health plan that provides health benefits solely through an insurance contract with a health insurance issuer or HMO, and that creates or receives protected health information in addition to summary health information as defined in §164.504(a) or information on whether the individual is participating in the group health plan, or is enrolled in or has disenrolled from a health insurance issuer or HMO offered by the plan, must:

(A) Maintain a notice under this section; and

(B) Provide such notice upon request to any person. The provisions of paragraph (c)(1) of this section do not apply to such group health plan.

(iii) A group health plan that provides health benefits solely through an insurance contract with a health insurance issuer or HMO, and does not create or receive protected health information other than summary health information as defined in §164.504(a) or information on whether an individual is participating in the group health plan, or is enrolled in or has disenrolled from a health insurance issuer or HMO offered by the plan, is not required to maintain or provide a notice under this section.

(3) Exception for inmates. An inmate does not have a right to notice under this section, and the requirements of this section do not apply to a correctional institution that is a covered entity.

(b) Implementation specifications: content of notice.

(1) Required elements. The covered entity must provide a notice that is written in plain language and that contains the elements required by this paragraph.

(i) Header. The notice must contain the following statement as a header or otherwise prominently displayed: "THIS NOTICE DESCRIBES HOW MEDICAL INFORMATION ABOUT YOU MAY BE USED AND DISCLOSED AND HOW YOU CAN GET ACCESS TO THIS INFORMATION. PLEASE REVIEW IT CAREFULLY."

(ii) Uses and disclosures. The notice must contain:

(A) A description, including at least one example, of the types of uses and disclosures that the covered entity is permitted by this subpart to make for each of the following purposes: treatment, payment, and health care operations.

(B) A description of each of the other purposes for which the covered entity is permitted or required by this subpart to use or disclose protected health information without the individual's written authorization.

(C) If a use or disclosure for any purpose described in paragraphs (b)(1)(ii)(A) or (B) of this section is prohibited or materially limited by other applicable law, the description of such use or disclosure must reflect the more stringent law as defined in §160.202.

(D) For each purpose described in paragraph (b)(1)(ii)(A) or (B) of this section, the description must include sufficient detail to place the individual on notice of the uses and disclosures that are permitted or required by this subpart and other applicable law.

(E) A statement that other uses and disclosures will be made only with the individual's written authorization and that the individual may revoke such authorization as provided by §164.508(b)(5).

(iii) Separate statements for certain uses or disclosures. If the covered entity intends to engage in any of the following activities, the description required by paragraph (b)(1)(ii)(A) of this section must include a separate statement, as applicable, that:

(A) The covered entity may contact the individual to provide appointment reminders or information about treatment alternatives or other heath-related benefits and services that may be of interest to the individual;

(B) The covered entity may contact the individual to raise funds for the covered entity; or

(C) A group health plan, or a health insurance issuer or HMO with respect to a group health plan, may disclose protected health information to the sponsor of the plan.

(iv) Individual rights. The notice must contain a statement of the individual's rights with respect to protected health information and a brief description of how the individual may exercise these rights, as follows:

(A) The right to request restrictions on certain uses and disclosures of protected health information as provided by §164.522(a), including a statement that the covered entity is not required to agree to a requested restriction;

(B) The right to receive confidential communications of protected health information as provided by §164.522(b), as applicable;

(C) The right to inspect and copy protected health information as provided by §164.524;

(D) The right to amend protected health information as provided by §164.526;

(E) The right to receive an accounting of disclosures of protected health information as provided by §164.528; and

(F) The right of an individual, including an individual who has agreed to receive the notice electronically in accordance with paragraph (c)(3) of this section, to obtain a paper copy of the notice from the covered entity upon request.

(v) Covered entity's duties. The notice must contain:

(A) A statement that the covered entity is required by law to maintain the privacy of protected health information and to provide individuals with notice of its legal duties and privacy practices with respect to protected health information;

(B) A statement that the covered entity is required to abide by the terms of the notice currently in effect; and

(C) For the covered entity to apply a change in a privacy practice that is described in the notice to protected health information that the covered entity created or received prior to issuing a revised notice, in accordance with §164.530(i)(2)(ii), a statement that it reserves the right to change the terms of its notice and to make the new notice provisions effective for all protected health information that it maintains. The statement must also describe how it will provide individuals with a revised notice.

(vi) Complaints. The notice must contain a statement that individuals may complain to the covered entity and to the Secretary if they believe their privacy rights have been violated, a brief description of how the individual may file a complaint with the covered entity, and a statement that the individual will not be retaliated against for filing a complaint.

(vii) Contact. The notice must contain the name, or title, and telephone number of a person or office to contact for further information as required by §164.530(a)(1)(ii).

(viii) Effective date. The notice must contain the date on which the notice is first in effect, which may not be earlier than the date on which the notice is printed or otherwise published.

(2) Optional elements.

(i) In addition to the information required by paragraph (b)(1) of this section, if a covered entity elects to limit the uses or disclosures that it is permitted to make under this subpart, the covered entity may describe its more limited uses or disclosures in its notice, provided that the covered entity may not include in its notice a limitation affecting its right to make a use or disclosure that is required by law or permitted by §164.512(j)(1)(i).

(ii) For the covered entity to apply a change in its more limited uses and disclosures to protected health information created or received prior to issuing a revised notice, in accordance with §164.530(i)(2)(ii), the notice must include the statements required by paragraph (b)(1)(v)(C) of this section.

(3) Revisions to the notice. The covered entity must promptly revise and distribute its notice whenever there is a material change to the uses or disclosures, the individual's rights, the covered entity's legal duties, or other privacy practices stated in the notice. Except when required by law, a material change to any term of the notice may not be implemented prior to the effective date of the notice in which such material change is reflected.

(c) Implementation specifications: provision of notice. A covered entity must make the notice required by this section available on request to any person and to individuals as specified in paragraphs (c)(1) through (c)(3) of this section, as applicable.

(1) Specific requirements for health plans.

(i) A health plan must provide notice:

(A) No later than the compliance date for the health plan, to individuals then covered by the plan;

(B) Thereafter, at the time of enrollment, to individuals who are new enrollees; and

(C) Within 60 days of a material revision to the notice, to individuals then covered by the plan.

(ii) No less frequently than once every three years, the health plan must notify individuals then covered by the plan of the availability of the notice and how to obtain the notice.

(iii) The health plan satisfies the requirements of paragraph (c)(1) of this section if notice is provided to the named insured of a policy under which coverage is provided to the named insured and one or more dependents.

(iv) If a health plan has more than one notice, it satisfies the requirements of paragraph (c)(1) of this section by providing the notice that is relevant to the individual or other person requesting the notice.

(2) Specific requirements for certain covered health care providers. A covered health care provider that has a direct treatment relationship with an individual must:

(i) Provide the notice:

(A) No later than the date of the first service delivery, including service delivered electronically, to such individual after the compliance date for the covered health care provider; or

(B) In an emergency treatment situation, as soon as reasonably practicable after the emergency treatment situation.

(ii) Except in an emergency treatment situation, make a good faith effort to obtain a written acknowledgment of receipt of the notice provided in accordance with paragraph (c)(2)(i) of this section, and if not obtained, document its good faith efforts to obtain such acknowledgment and the reason why the acknowledgment was not obtained;

(iii) If the covered health care provider maintains a physical service delivery site:

(A) Have the notice available at the service delivery site for individuals to request to take with them; and

(B) Post the notice in a clear and prominent location where it is reasonable to expect individuals seeking service from the covered health care provider to be able to read the notice; and

(iv) Whenever the notice is revised, make the notice available upon request on or after the effective date of the revision and promptly comply with the requirements of paragraph (c)(2)(iii) of this section, if applicable.

(3) Specific requirements for electronic notice.

(i) A covered entity that maintains a web site that provides information about the covered entity's customer services or benefits must prominently post its notice on the web site and make the notice available electronically through the web site.

(ii) A covered entity may provide the notice required by this section to an individual by e-mail, if the individual agrees to electronic notice and such agreement has not been withdrawn. If the covered entity knows that the e-mail transmission has failed, a paper copy of the notice must be provided to the individual. Provision of electronic notice by the covered entity will satisfy the provision requirements of paragraph (c) of this section when timely made in accordance with paragraph (c)(1) or (2) of this section.

(iii) For purposes of paragraph (c)(2)(i) of this section, if the first service delivery to an individual is delivered electronically, the covered health care provider must provide electronic notice automatically and contemporaneously in response to the individual's first request for service. The requirements in paragraph (c)(2)(ii) of this section apply to electronic notice.

(iv) The individual who is the recipient of electronic notice retains the right to obtain a paper copy of the notice from a covered entity upon request.

(d) Implementation specifications: joint notice by separate covered entities. Covered entities that participate in organized health care arrangements may comply with this section by a joint notice, provided that:

(1) The covered entities participating in the organized health care arrangement agree to abide by the terms of the notice with respect to protected health information created or received by the covered entity as part of its participation in the organized health care arrangement;

(2) The joint notice meets the implementation specifications in paragraph (b) of this section, except that the statements required by this section may be altered to reflect the fact that the notice covers more than one covered entity; and

(i) Describes with reasonable specificity the covered entities, or class of entities, to which the joint notice applies;

(ii) Describes with reasonable specificity the service delivery sites, or classes of service delivery sites, to which the joint notice applies; and

(iii) If applicable, states that the covered entities participating in the organized health care arrangement will share protected health information with each other, as necessary to carry out treatment, payment, or health care operations relating to the organized health care arrangement.

(3) The covered entities included in the joint notice must provide the notice to individuals in accordance with the applicable implementation specifications of paragraph (c) of this section. Provision of the joint notice to an individual by any one of the covered entities included in the joint notice will satisfy the provision requirement of paragraph (c) of this section with respect to all others covered by the joint notice.

(e) Implementation specifications: Documentation. A covered entity must document compliance with the notice requirements, as required by §164.530(j), by retaining copies of the notices issued by the covered entity and, if applicable, any written acknowledgments of receipt of the notice or documentation of good faith efforts to obtain such written acknowledgment, in accordance with paragraph (c)(2)(ii) of this section.

§164.522 Rights to request privacy protection for protected health information.

(a)(1) Standard: right of an individual to request restriction of uses and disclosures.

(i) A covered entity must permit an individual to request that the covered entity restrict:

(A) Uses or disclosures of protected health information about the individual to carry out treatment, payment, or health care operations; and

(B) Disclosures permitted under §164.510(b).

(ii) A covered entity is not required to agree to a restriction.

(iii) A covered entity that agrees to a restriction under paragraph (a)(1)(i) of this section may not use or disclose protected health information in violation of such restriction, except that, if the individual who requested the restriction is in need of emergency treatment and the restricted protected health information is needed to provide the emergency treatment, the covered entity may use the restricted protected health information, or may disclose such information to a health care provider, to provide such treatment to the individual.

(iv) If restricted protected health information is disclosed to a health care provider for emergency treatment under paragraph (a)(1)(iii) of this section, the covered entity must request that such health care provider not further use or disclose the information.

(v) A restriction agreed to by a covered entity under paragraph (a) of this section, is not effective under this subpart to prevent uses or disclosures permitted or required under §§164.502(a)(2)(ii), 164.510(a) or 164.512.

(2) Implementation specifications: terminating a restriction. A covered entity may terminate its agreement to a restriction, if:

(i) The individual agrees to or requests the termination in writing;

(ii) The individual orally agrees to the termination and the oral agreement is documented; or

(iii) The covered entity informs the individual that it is terminating its agreement to a restriction, except that such termination is only effective with respect to protected health information created or received after it has so informed the individual.

(3) Implementation specification: documentation. A covered entity that agrees to a restriction must document the restriction in accordance with §164.530(j).

(b)(1) Standard: confidential communications requirements.

(i) A covered health care provider must permit individuals to request and must accommodate reasonable requests by individuals to receive communications of protected health information from the covered health care provider by alternative means or at alternative locations.

(ii) A health plan must permit individuals to request and must accommodate reasonable requests by individuals to receive communications of protected health information from the health plan by alternative means or at alternative locations, if the individual clearly states that the disclosure of all or part of that information could endanger the individual.

(2) Implementation specifications: conditions on providing confidential communications.

(i) A covered entity may require the individual to make a request for a confidential communication described in paragraph (b)(1) of this section in writing.

(ii) A covered entity may condition the provision of a reasonable accommodation on:

(A) When appropriate, information as to how payment, if any, will be handled; and

(B) Specification of an alternative address or other method of contact.

(iii) A covered health care provider may not require an explanation from the individual as to the basis for the request as a condition of providing communications on a confidential basis.

(iv) A health plan may require that a request contain a statement that disclosure of all or part of the information to which the request pertains could endanger the individual.

§164.524 Access of individuals to protected health information.

(a) Standard: access to protected health information.

(1) Right of access. Except as otherwise provided in paragraph (a)(2) or (a)(3) of this section, an individual has a right of access to inspect and obtain a copy of protected health information about the individual in a designated record set, for as long as the protected health information is maintained in the designated record set, except for:

(i) Psychotherapy notes;

(ii) Information compiled in reasonable anticipation of, or for use in, a civil, criminal, or administrative action or proceeding; and

(iii) Protected health information maintained by a covered entity that is:

(A) Subject to the Clinical Laboratory Improvements Amendments of 1988, 42 U.S.C. 263a, to the extent the provision of access to the individual would be prohibited by law; or

(B) Exempt from the Clinical Laboratory Improvements Amendments of 1988, pursuant to 42 CFR 493.3(a)(2).

(2) Unreviewable grounds for denial. A covered entity may deny an individual access without providing the individual an opportunity for review, in the following circumstances.

(i) The protected health information is excepted from the right of access by paragraph (a)(1) of this section.

(ii) A covered entity that is a correctional institution or a covered health care provider acting under the direction of the correctional institution may deny, in whole or in part, an inmate's request to obtain a copy of protected health information, if obtaining such copy would jeopardize the health, safety, security, custody, or rehabilitation of the individual or of other inmates, or the safety of any officer, employee, or other person at the correctional institution or responsible for the transporting of the inmate.

(iii) An individual's access to protected health information created or obtained by a covered health care provider in the course of research that includes treatment may be temporarily suspended for as long as the research is in progress, provided that the individual has agreed to the denial of access when consenting to participate in the research that includes treatment, and the covered health care provider has informed the individual that the right of access will be reinstated upon completion of the research.

(iv) An individual's access to protected health information that is contained in records that are subject to the Privacy Act, 5 U.S.C. §552a, may be denied, if the denial of access under the Privacy Act would meet the requirements of that law.

(v) An individual's access may be denied if the protected health information was obtained from someone other than a health care provider under a promise of confidentiality and the access requested would be reasonably likely to reveal the source of the information.

(3) Reviewable grounds for denial. A covered entity may deny an individual access, provided that the individual is given a right to have such denials reviewed, as required by paragraph (a)(4) of this section, in the following circumstances:

(i) A licensed health care professional has determined, in the exercise of professional judgment, that the access requested is reasonably likely to endanger the life or physical safety of the individual or another person;

(ii) The protected health information makes reference to another person (unless such other person is a health care provider) and a licensed health care professional has determined, in the exercise of professional judgment, that the access requested is reasonably likely to cause substantial harm to such other person; or

(iii) The request for access is made by the individual's personal representative and a licensed health care professional has determined, in the exercise of professional judgment, that the provision of access to such personal representative is reasonably likely to cause substantial harm to the individual or another person.

(4) Review of a denial of access. If access is denied on a ground permitted under paragraph (a)(3) of this section, the individual has the right to have the denial reviewed by a licensed health care professional who is designated by the covered entity to act as a reviewing official and who did not participate in the original decision to deny. The covered entity must provide or deny access in accordance with the determination of the reviewing official under paragraph (d)(4) of this section.

(b) Implementation specifications: requests for access and timely action.

(1) Individual's request for access. The covered entity must permit an individual to request access to inspect or to obtain a copy of the protected health information about the individual that is maintained in a designated record set. The covered entity may require individuals to make requests for access in writing, provided that it informs individuals of such a requirement.

(2) Timely action by the covered entity.

(i) Except as provided in paragraph (b)(2)(ii) of this section, the covered entity must act on a request for access no later than 30 days after receipt of the request as follows.

(A) If the covered entity grants the request, in whole or in part, it must inform the individual of the acceptance of the request and provide the access requested, in accordance with paragraph (c) of this section.

(B) If the covered entity denies the request, in whole or in part, it must provide the individual with a written denial, in accordance with paragraph (d) of this section.

(ii) If the request for access is for protected health information that is not maintained or accessible to the covered entity on-site, the covered entity must take an action required by paragraph (b)(2)(i) of this section by no later than 60 days from the receipt of such a request.

(iii) If the covered entity is unable to take an action required by paragraph (b)(2)(i)(A) or (B) of this section within the time required by paragraph (b)(2)(i) or (ii) of this section, as applicable, the covered entity may extend the time for such actions by no more than 30 days, provided that:

(A) The covered entity, within the time limit set by paragraph (b)(2)(i) or (ii) of this section, as applicable, provides the individual with a written statement of the reasons for the delay and the date by which the covered entity will complete its action on the request; and

(B) The covered entity may have only one such extension of time for action on a request for access.

(c) Implementation specifications: provision of access. If the covered entity provides an individual with access, in whole or in part, to protected health information, the covered entity must comply with the following requirements.

(1) Providing the access requested. The covered entity must provide the access requested by individuals, including inspection or obtaining a copy, or both, of the protected health information about them in designated record sets. If the same protected health information that is the subject of a request for access is maintained in more than one designated record set or at more than one location, the covered entity need only produce the protected health information once in response to a request for access.

(2) Form of access requested.

(i) The covered entity must provide the individual with access to the protected health information in the form or format requested by the individual, if it is readily producible in such form or format; or, if not, in a readable hard copy form or such other form or format as agreed to by the covered entity and the individual.

(ii) The covered entity may provide the individual with a summary of the protected health information requested, in lieu of providing access to the protected health information or may provide an explanation of the protected health information to which access has been provided, if:

(A) The individual agrees in advance to such a summary or explanation; and

(B) The individual agrees in advance to the fees imposed, if any, by the covered entity for such summary or explanation.

(3) Time and manner of access. The covered entity must provide the access as requested by the individual in a timely manner as required by paragraph (b)(2) of this section, including arranging with the individual for a convenient time and place to inspect or obtain a copy of the protected health information, or mailing the copy of the protected health information at the individual's request. The covered entity may discuss the scope, format, and other aspects of the request for access with the individual as necessary to facilitate the timely provision of access.

(4) Fees. If the individual requests a copy of the protected health information or agrees to a summary or explanation of such information, the covered entity may impose a reasonable, cost-based fee, provided that the fee includes only the cost of:

(i) Copying, including the cost of supplies for and labor of copying, the protected health information requested by the individual;

(ii) Postage, when the individual has requested the copy, or the summary or explanation, be mailed; and

(iii) Preparing an explanation or summary of the protected health information, if agreed to by the individual as required by paragraph (c)(2)(ii) of this section.

(d) Implementation specifications: denial of access. If the covered entity denies access, in whole or in part, to protected health information, the covered entity must comply with the following requirements.

(1) Making other information accessible. The covered entity must, to the extent possible, give the individual access to any other protected health information requested, after excluding the protected health information as to which the covered entity has a ground to deny access.

(2) Denial. The covered entity must provide a timely, written denial to the individual, in accordance with paragraph (b)(2) of this section. The denial must be in plain language and contain:

(i) The basis for the denial;

(ii) If applicable, a statement of the individual's review rights under paragraph (a)(4) of this section, including a description of how the individual may exercise such review rights; and

(iii) A description of how the individual may complain to the covered entity pursuant to the complaint procedures in §164.530(d) or to the Secretary pursuant to the procedures in §160.306. The description must include the name, or title, and telephone number of the contact person or office designated in §164.530(a)(1)(ii).

(3) Other responsibility. If the covered entity does not maintain the protected health information that is the subject of the individual's request for access, and the covered entity knows where the requested information is maintained, the covered entity must inform the individual where to direct the request for access.

(4) Review of denial requested. If the individual has requested a review of a denial under paragraph (a)(4) of this section, the covered entity must designate a licensed health care professional, who was not directly involved in the denial to review the decision to deny access. The covered entity must promptly refer a request for review to such designated reviewing official. The designated reviewing official must determine, within a reasonable period of time, whether or not to deny the access requested based on the standards in paragraph (a)(3) of this section. The covered entity must promptly provide written notice to the individual of the determination of the designated reviewing official and take other action as required by this section to carry out the designated reviewing official's determination.

(e) Implementation specification: documentation. A covered entity must document the following and retain the documentation as required by §164.530(j):

(1) The designated record sets that are subject to access by individuals; and

(2) The titles of the persons or offices responsible for receiving and processing requests for access by individuals.

§164.526 Amendment of protected health information.

(a) Standard: right to amend.

(1) Right to amend. An individual has the right to have a covered entity amend protected health information or a record about the individual in a designated record set for as long as the protected health information is maintained in the designated record set.

(2) Denial of amendment. A covered entity may deny an individual's request for amendment, if it determines that the protected health information or record that is the subject of the request:

(i) Was not created by the covered entity, unless the individual provides a reasonable basis to believe that the originator of protected health information is no longer available to act on the requested amendment;

(ii) Is not part of the designated record set;

(iii) Would not be available for inspection under §164.524; or

(iv) Is accurate and complete.

(b) Implementation specifications: requests for amendment and timely action.

(1) Individual's request for amendment. The covered entity must permit an individual to request that the covered entity amend the protected health information maintained in the designated record set. The covered entity may require individuals to make requests for amendment in writing and to provide a reason to support a requested amendment, provided that it informs individuals in advance of such requirements.

(2) Timely action by the covered entity.

(i) The covered entity must act on the individual's request for an amendment no later than 60 days after receipt of such a request, as follows.

(A) If the covered entity grants the requested amendment, in whole or in part, it must take the actions required by paragraphs (c)(1) and (2) of this section.

(B) If the covered entity denies the requested amendment, in whole or in part, it must provide the individual with a written denial, in accordance with paragraph (d)(1) of this section.

(ii) If the covered entity is unable to act on the amendment within the time required by paragraph (b)(2)(i) of this section, the covered entity may extend the time for such action by no more than 30 days, provided that:

(A) The covered entity, within the time limit set by paragraph (b)(2)(i) of this section, provides the individual with a written statement of the reasons for the delay and the date by which the covered entity will complete its action on the request; and

(B) The covered entity may have only one such extension of time for action on a request for an amendment.

(c) Implementation specifications: accepting the amendment. If the covered entity accepts the requested amendment, in whole or in part, the covered entity must comply with the following requirements.

(1) Making the amendment. The covered entity must make the appropriate amendment to the protected health information or record that is the subject of the request for amendment by, at a minimum, identifying the records in the designated record set that are affected by the amendment and appending or otherwise providing a link to the location of the amendment.

(2) Informing the individual. In accordance with paragraph (b) of this section, the covered entity must timely inform the individual that the amendment is accepted and obtain the individual's identification of and agreement to have the covered entity notify the relevant persons with which the amendment needs to be shared in accordance with paragraph (c)(3) of this section.

(3) Informing others. The covered entity must make reasonable efforts to inform and provide the amendment within a reasonable time to:

(i) Persons identified by the individual as having received protected health information about the individual and needing the amendment; and

(ii) Persons, including business associates, that the covered entity knows have the protected health information that is the subject of the amendment and that may have relied, or could foreseeably rely, on such information to the detriment of the individual.

(d) Implementation specifications: denying the amendment. If the covered entity denies the requested amendment, in whole or in part, the covered entity must comply with the following requirements.

(1) Denial. The covered entity must provide the individual with a timely, written denial, in accordance with paragraph (b)(2) of this section. The denial must use plain language and contain:

(i) The basis for the denial, in accordance with paragraph (a)(2) of this section;

(ii) The individual's right to submit a written statement disagreeing with the denial and how the individual may file such a statement;

(iii) A statement that, if the individual does not submit a statement of disagreement, the individual may request that the covered entity provide the individual's request for amendment and the denial with any future disclosures of the protected health information that is the subject of the amendment; and

(iv) A description of how the individual may complain to the covered entity pursuant to the complaint procedures established in §164.530(d) or to the Secretary pursuant to the procedures established in §160.306. The description must include the name, or title, and telephone number of the contact person or office designated in §164.530(a)(1)(ii).

(2) Statement of disagreement. The covered entity must permit the individual to. submit to the covered entity a written statement disagreeing with the denial of all or part of a requested amendment and the basis of such disagreement. The covered entity may reasonably limit the length of a statement of disagreement.

(3) Rebuttal statement. The covered entity may prepare a written rebuttal to the individual's statement of disagreement. Whenever such a rebuttal is prepared, the covered entity must provide a copy to the individual who submitted the statement of disagreement.

(4) Recordkeeping. The covered entity must, as appropriate, identify the record or protected health information in the designated record set that is the subject of the disputed amendment and append or otherwise link the individual's request for an amendment, the covered entity's denial of the request, the individual's statement of disagreement, if any, and the covered entity's rebuttal, if any, to the designated record set.

(5) Future disclosures.

(i) If a statement of disagreement has been submitted by the individual, the covered entity must include the material appended in accordance with paragraph (d)(4) of this section, or, at the election of the covered entity, an accurate summary of any such information, with any subsequent disclosure of the protected health information to which the disagreement relates.

(ii) If the individual has not submitted a written statement of disagreement, the covered entity must include the individual's request for amendment and its denial, or an accurate summary of such information, with any subsequent disclosure of the protected health information only if the individual has requested such action in accordance with paragraph (d)(1)(iii) of this section.

(iii) When a subsequent disclosure described in paragraph (d)(5)(i) or (ii) of this section is made using a standard transaction under part 162 of this subchapter that does not permit the additional material to be included with the disclosure, the covered entity may separately transmit the material required by paragraph (d)(5)(i) or (ii) of this section, as applicable, to the recipient of the standard transaction.

(e) Implementation specification: actions on notices of amendment. A covered entity that is informed by another covered entity of an amendment to an individual's protected health information, in accordance with paragraph (c)(3) of this section, must amend the protected health information in designated record sets as provided by paragraph (c)(1) of this section.

(f) Implementation specification: documentation. A covered entity must document the titles of the persons or offices responsible for receiving and processing requests for amendments by individuals and retain the documentation as required by §164.530(j).

§164.528 Accounting of disclosures of protected health information.

(a) Standard: right to an accounting of disclosures of protected health information.

(1) An individual has a right to receive an accounting of disclosures of protected health information made by a covered entity in the six years prior to the date on which the accounting is requested, except for disclosures:

(i) To carry out treatment, payment and health care operations as provided in §164.506;

(ii) To individuals of protected health information about them as provided in §164.502;

(iii) Incident to a use or disclosure otherwise permitted or required by this subpart, as provided in §164.502;

(iv) Pursuant to an authorization as provided in §164.508;

(v) For the facility's directory or to persons involved in the individual's care or other notification purposes as provided in §164.510;

(vi) For national security or intelligence purposes as provided in §164.512(k)(2);

(vii) To correctional institutions or law enforcement officials as provided in §164.512(k)(5);

(viii) As part of a limited data set in accordance with §164.514(e); or

(ix) That occurred prior to the compliance date for the covered entity.

(2) (i) The covered entity must temporarily suspend an individual's right to receive an accounting of disclosures to a health oversight agency or law enforcement official, as provided in §164.512(d) or (f), respectively, for the time specified by such agency or official, if such agency or official provides the covered entity with a written statement that such an accounting to the individual would be reasonably likely to impede the agency's activities and specifying the time for which such a suspension is required.

(ii) If the agency or official statement in paragraph (a)(2)(i) of this section is made orally, the covered entity must:

(A) Document the statement, including the identity of the agency or official making the statement;

(B) Temporarily suspend the individual's right to an accounting of disclosures subject to the statement; and

(C) Limit the temporary suspension to no longer than 30 days from the date of the oral statement, unless a written statement pursuant to paragraph (a)(2)(i) of this section is submitted during that time.

(3) An individual may request an accounting of disclosures for a period of time less than six years from the date of the request.

(b) Implementation specifications: content of the accounting. The covered entity must provide the individual with a written accounting that meets the following requirements.

(1) Except as otherwise provided by paragraph (a) of this section, the accounting must include disclosures of protected health information that occurred during the six years (or such shorter time period at the request of the individual as provided in paragraph (a)(3) of this section) prior to the date of the request for an accounting, including disclosures to or by business associates of the covered entity.

(2) Except as otherwise provided by paragraphs (b)(3) or (b)(4) of this section, the accounting must include for each disclosure:

(i) The date of the disclosure;

(ii) The name of the entity or person who received the protected health information and, if known, the address of such entity or person;

(iii) A brief description of the protected health information disclosed; and

(iv) A brief statement of the purpose of the disclosure that reasonably informs the individual of the basis for the disclosure or, in lieu of such statement, a copy of a written request for a disclosure under §§164.502(a)(2)(ii) or 164.512, if any.

(3) If, during the period covered by the accounting, the covered entity has made multiple disclosures of protected health information to the same person or entity for a single purpose under §§164.502(a)(2)(ii) or 164.512, the accounting may, with respect to such multiple disclosures, provide:

(i) The information required by paragraph (b)(2) of this section for the first disclosure during the accounting period;

(ii) The frequency, periodicity, or number of the disclosures made during the accounting period; and

(iii) The date of the last such disclosure during the accounting period.

(4) (i) If, during the period covered by the accounting, the covered entity has made disclosures of protected health information for a particular research purpose in accordance with §164.512(i) for 50 or more individuals, the accounting may, with respect to such disclosures for which the protected health information about the individual may have been included, provide:

(A) The name of the protocol or other research activity;

(B) A description, in plain language, of the research protocol or other research activity, including the purpose of the research and the criteria for selecting particular records;

(C) A brief description of the type of protected health information that was disclosed;

(D) The date or period of time during which such disclosures occurred, or may have occurred, including the date of the last such disclosure during the accounting period;

(E) The name, address, and telephone number of the entity that sponsored the research and of the researcher to whom the information was disclosed; and

(F) A statement that the protected health information of the individual may or may not have been disclosed for a particular protocol or other research activity.

(ii) If the covered entity provides an accounting for research disclosures, in accordance with paragraph (b)(4) of this section, and if it is reasonably likely that the protected health information of the individual was disclosed for such research protocol or activity, the covered entity shall, at the request of the individual, assist in contacting the entity that sponsored the research and the researcher.

(c) Implementation specifications: provision of the accounting.

(1) The covered entity must act on the individual's request for an accounting, no later than 60 days after receipt of such a request, as follows.

(i) The covered entity must provide the individual with the accounting requested; or

(ii) If the covered entity is unable to provide the accounting within the time required by paragraph (c)(1) of this section, the covered entity may extend the time to provide the accounting by no more than 30 days, provided that::

(A) The covered entity, within the time limit set by paragraph (c)(1) of this section, provides the individual with a written statement of the reasons for the delay and the date by which the covered entity will provide the accounting; and

(B) The covered entity may have only one such extension of time for action on a request for an accounting.

(2) The covered entity must provide the first accounting to an individual in any 12 month period without charge. The covered entity may impose a reasonable, cost-based fee for each subsequent request for an accounting by the same individual within the 12 month period, provided that the covered entity informs the individual in advance of the fee and provides the individual with an opportunity to withdraw or modify the request for a subsequent accounting in order to avoid or reduce the fee.

(d) Implementation specification: documentation. A covered entity must document the following and retain the documentation as required by §164.530(j):

(1) The information required to be included in an accounting under paragraph (b) of this section for disclosures of protected health information that are subject to an accounting under paragraph (a) of this section;

(2) The written accounting that is provided to the individual under this section; and

(3) The titles of the persons or offices responsible for receiving and processing requests for an accounting by individuals.

§164.530 Administrative requirements.

(a)(1) Standard: personnel designations.

(i) A covered entity must designate a privacy official who is responsible for the development and implementation of the policies and procedures of the entity.

(ii) A covered entity must designate a contact person or office who is responsible for receiving complaints under this section and who is able to provide further information about matters covered by the notice required by §164.520.

(2) Implementation specification: personnel designations. A covered entity must document the personnel designations in paragraph (a)(1) of this section as required by paragraph (j) of this section.

(b)(1) Standard: training. A covered entity must train all members of its workforce on the policies and procedures with respect to protected health information required by this subpart, as necessary and appropriate for the members of the workforce to carry out their function within the covered entity.

(2) Implementation specifications: training.

(i) A covered entity must provide training that meets the requirements of paragraph (b)(1) of this section, as follows:

(A) To each member of the covered entity's workforce by no later than the compliance date for the covered entity;

(B) Thereafter, to each new member of the workforce within a reasonable period of time after the person joins the covered entity's workforce; and

(C) To each member of the covered entity's workforce whose functions are affected by a material change in the policies or procedures required by this subpart, within a reasonable period of time after the material change becomes effective in accordance with paragraph (i) of this section.

(ii) A covered entity must document that the training as described in paragraph (b)(2)(i) of this section has been provided, as required by paragraph (j) of this section.

(c)(1) Standard: safeguards. A covered entity must have in place appropriate administrative, technical, and physical safeguards to protect the privacy of protected health information.

(2) Implementation specification: safeguards.

(i) A covered entity must reasonably safeguard protected health information from any intentional or unintentional use or disclosure that is in violation of the standards, implementation specifications or other requirements of this subpart.

(ii) A covered entity must reasonably safeguard protected health information to limit incidental uses or disclosures made pursuant to an otherwise permitted or required use or disclosure.

(d)(1) Standard: complaints to the covered entity. A covered entity must provide a process for individuals to make complaints concerning the covered entity's policies and procedures required by this subpart or its compliance with such policies and procedures or the requirements of this subpart.

(2) Implementation specification: documentation of complaints. As required by paragraph (j) of this section, a covered entity must document all complaints received, and their disposition, if any.

(e)(1) Standard: sanctions. A covered entity must have and apply appropriate sanctions against members of its workforce who fail to comply with the privacy policies and procedures of the covered entity or the requirements of this subpart. This standard does not apply to a member of the covered entity's workforce with respect to actions that are covered by and that meet the conditions of §164.502(j) or paragraph (g)(2) of this section.

(2) Implementation specification: documentation. As required by paragraph (j) of this section, a covered entity must document the sanctions that are applied, if any.

(f) Standard: mitigation. A covered entity must mitigate, to the extent practicable, any harmful effect that is known to the covered entity of a use or disclosure of protected health information in violation of its policies and procedures or the requirements of this subpart by the covered entity or its business associate.

(g) Standard: refraining from intimidating or retaliatory acts. A covered entity may not intimidate, threaten, coerce, discriminate against, or take other retaliatory action against:

(1) Individuals. Any individual for the exercise by the individual of any right under, or for participation by the individual in any process established by this subpart, including the filing of a complaint under this section;

(2) Individuals and others. Any individual or other person for:

(i) Filing of a complaint with the Secretary under subpart C of part 160 of this subchapter;

(ii) Testifying, assisting, or participating in an investigation, compliance review, proceeding, or hearing under Part C of Title XI; or

(iii) Opposing any act or practice made unlawful by this subpart, provided the individual or person has a good faith belief that the practice opposed is unlawful, and the manner of the opposition is reasonable and does not involve a disclosure of protected health information in violation of this subpart.

(h) Standard: waiver of rights. A covered entity may not require individuals to waive their rights under §160.306 of this subchapter or this subpart as a condition of the provision of treatment, payment, enrollment in a health plan, or eligibility for benefits.

(i)(1) Standard: policies and procedures. A covered entity must implement policies and procedures with respect to protected health information that are designed to comply with the standards, implementation specifications, or other requirements of this subpart. The policies and procedures must be reasonably designed, taking into account the size of and the type of activities that relate to protected health information undertaken by the covered entity, to ensure such compliance. This standard is not to be construed to permit or excuse an action that violates any other standard, implementation specification, or other requirement of this subpart.

(2) Standard: changes to policies or procedures.

(i) A covered entity must change its policies and procedures as necessary and appropriate to comply with changes in the law, including the standards, requirements, and implementation specifications of this subpart;

(ii) When a covered entity changes a privacy practice that is stated in the notice described in §164.520, and makes corresponding changes to its policies and procedures, it may make the changes effective for protected health information that it created or received prior to the effective date of the notice revision, if the covered entity has, in accordance with §164.520(b)(1)(v)(C), included in the notice a statement reserving its right to make such a change in its privacy practices; or

(iii) A covered entity may make any other changes to policies and procedures at any time, provided that the changes are documented and implemented in accordance with paragraph (i)(5) of this section.

(3) Implementation specification: changes in law. Whenever there is a change in law that necessitates a change to the covered entity's policies or procedures, the covered entity must promptly document and implement the revised policy or procedure. If the change in law materially affects the content of the notice required by §164.520, the covered entity must promptly make the appropriate revisions to the notice in accordance with §164.520(b)(3). Nothing in this paragraph may be used by a covered entity to excuse a failure to comply with the law.

(4) Implementation specifications: changes to privacy practices stated in the notice.

(i) To implement a change as provided by paragraph (i)(2)(ii) of this section, a covered entity must:

(A) Ensure that the policy or procedure, as revised to reflect a change in the covered entity's privacy practice as stated in its notice, complies with the standards, requirements, and implementation specifications of this subpart;

(B) Document the policy or procedure, as revised, as required by paragraph (j) of this section; and

(C) Revise the notice as required by §164.520(b)(3) to state the changed practice and make the revised notice available as required by §164.520(c). The covered entity may not implement a change to a policy or procedure prior to the effective date of the revised notice.

(ii) If a covered entity has not reserved its right under §164.520(b)(1)(v)(C) to change a privacy practice that is stated in the notice, the covered entity is bound by the privacy practices as stated in the notice with respect to protected health information created or received while such notice is in effect. A covered entity may change a privacy practice that is stated in the notice, and the related policies and procedures, without having reserved the right to do so, provided that:

(A) Such change meets the implementation specifications in paragraphs (i)(4)(i)(A)-(C) of this section; and

(B) Such change is effective only with respect to protected health information created or received after the effective date of the notice.

(5) Implementation specification: changes to other policies or procedures. A covered entity may change, at any time, a policy or procedure that does not materially affect the content of the notice required by §164.520, provided that:

(i) The policy or procedure, as revised, complies with the standards, requirements, and implementation specifications of this subpart; and

(ii) Prior to the effective date of the change, the policy or procedure, as revised, is documented as required by paragraph (j) of this section.

(j)(1) Standard: documentation. A covered entity must:

(i) Maintain the policies and procedures provided for in paragraph (i) of this section in written or electronic form;

(ii) If a communication is required by this subpart to be in writing, maintain such writing, or an electronic copy, as documentation; and

(iii) If an action, activity, or designation is required by this subpart to be documented, maintain a written or electronic record of such action, activity, or designation.

(2) Implementation specification: retention period. A covered entity must retain the documentation required by paragraph (j)(1) of this section for six years from the date of its creation or the date when it last was in effect, whichever is later.

(k) Standard: group health plans.

(1) A group health plan is not subject to the standards or implementation specifications in paragraphs (a) through (f) and (i) of this section, to the extent that:

(i) The group health plan provides health benefits solely through an insurance contract with a health insurance issuer or an HMO; and

(ii) The group health plan does not create or receive protected health information, except for:

(A) Summary health information as defined in §164.504(a); or

(B) Information on whether the individual is participating in the group health plan, or is enrolled in or has disenrolled from a health insurance issuer or HMO offered by the plan.

(2) A group health plan described in paragraph (k)(1) of this section is subject to the standard and implementation specification in paragraph (j) of this section only with respect to plan documents amended in accordance with §164.504(f). 225.116(d), 24 CFR 60.116(d), 28 CFR 46.116(d), 32 CFR 219.116(d), 34 CFR 97.116(d), 38 CFR 16.116(d), 40 CFR 26.116(d), 45 CFR 46.116(d), 45 CFR 690.116(d), or 49 CFR 11.116(d), provided that a covered entity must obtain authorization in accordance with §164.508 if, after the compliance date, informed and §§164.524, 164.526, 164.528, and 164.530(f) with respect to protected health information held by a business associate.

§164.532 Transition provisions.

(a) *Standard: Effect of prior authorizations.*

Notwithstanding §§164.508 and 164.512(i), a covered entity may use or disclose protected health information, consistent with paragraphs (b) and (c) of this section, pursuant to an authorization or other express legal permission obtained from an individual permitting the use or disclosure of protected health information, informed consent of the individual to participate in research, or a waiver of informed consent by an IRB.

(b) *Implementation specification: Effect of prior authorization for purposes other than research.*

Notwithstanding any provisions in §164.508, a covered entity may use or disclose protected health information that it created or received prior to the applicable compliance date of this subpart pursuant to an authorization or other express legal permission obtained from an individual prior to the applicable compliance date of this subpart, provided that the authorization or other express legal permission specifically permits such use or disclosure and there is no agreed-to restriction in accordance with § 164.522(a).

(c) *Implementation specification: Effect of prior permission for research.*

Notwithstanding any provisions in §§164.508 and 164.512(i), a covered entity may, to the extent allowed by one of the following permissions, use or disclose, for research, protected health information that it created or received either before or after the applicable compliance date of this subpart, provided that there is no agreed-to restriction in accordance with

§64.522(a), and the covered entity has obtained, prior to the applicable compliance date, either:

(1) An authorization or other express legal permission from an individual to use or disclose protected health information for the research;

(2) The informed consent of the individual to participate in the research; or

(3) A waiver, by an IRB, of informed consent for the research, in accordance with 7 CFR 1c.116(d), 10 CFR 745.116(d), 14 CFR 1230.116(d), 15 CFR 27.116(d), 16 CFR 1028.116(d), 21 CFR 50.24, 22 CFR 225.116(d), 24 CFR 60.116(d), 28 CFR 46.116(d), 32 CFR 219.116(d), 34 CFR 97.116(d), 38 CFR 16.116(d), 40 CFR 26.116(d), 45 CFR 46.116(d), 45 CFR 690.116(d), or 49 CFR 11.116(d), provided that a covered entity must obtain authorization in accordance with § 164.508 if, after the compliance date, informed consent is sought from an individual participating in the research.

(d) *Standard: Effect of prior contracts or other arrangements with business associates.*

Notwithstanding any other provisions of this subpart, a covered entity, other than a small health plan, may disclose protected health information to a business associate and may allow a business associate to create, receive, or use protected health information on its behalf pursuant to a written contract or other written arrangement with such business associate that does not comply with §§164.502(e) and 164.504(e) consistent with the requirements, and only for such time, set forth in paragraph (e) of this section.

(e) Implementation specification: Deemed compliance.

(1) Qualification. Notwithstanding other sections of this subpart, a covered entity, other than a small health plan, is deemed to be in compliance with the documentation and contract requirements of §§164.502(e) and 164.504(e), with respect to a particular business associate relationship, for the time period set forth in paragraph (e)(2) of this section, if:

(i) Prior to October 15, 2002, such covered entity has entered into and is operating pursuant to a written contract or other written arrangement with a business associate for such business associate to perform functions or activities or provide services that make the entity a business associate; and

(ii) The contract or other arrangement is not renewed or modified from October 15, 2002, until the compliance date set forth in §164.534.

(2) Limited deemed compliance period. A prior contract or other arrangement that meets the qualification requirements in paragraph (e) of this section, shall be deemed compliant until the earlier of:

(i) The date such contract or other arrangement is renewed or modified on or after the compliance date set forth in §164.534; or (ii) April 14, 2004.

(3) Covered entity responsibilities.

Nothing in this section shall alter the requirements of a covered entity to comply with Part 160, Subpart C of this subchapter and §§164.524, 164.526, 164.528, and 164.530(f) with respect to protected health information held by a business associate.

§164.534 Compliance dates for initial implementation of the privacy standards.

(a) Health care providers. A covered health care provider must comply with the applicable requirements of this subpart no later than April 14, 2003.

(b) Health plans. A health plan must comply with the applicable requirements of this subpart no later than the following date, as applicable:

(1) Health plans other than small health plans—April 14, 2003.

(2) Small health plans—April 14, 2004.

(c) Health care clearinghouses. A health care clearinghouse must comply with the applicable requirements of this subpart no later than April 14, 2003.

About CenterWatch

CenterWatch is a Boston-based publishing and information services company that focuses on the clinical trials industry. We provide a variety of information services used by pharmaceutical and biotechnology companies, CROs, SMOs and investigative sites involved in the management and conduct of clinical trials. CenterWatch also provides educational materials for clinical research professionals, health professionals and for health consumers. We provide market research and market intelligence services that many major companies have retained to help develop new business strategies, to guide the implementation of new clinical research-related initiatives and to assist in due diligence activities. Some of our top publications and services are described below. For a comprehensive listing with detailed information about our publications and services, please visit our web site at www.centerwatch.com. You can also contact us at (800) 765-9647 for subscription and order information.

22 Thomson Place · Boston, MA 02210
Phone (617) 856-5900 · Fax (617) 856-5901
www.centerwatch.com

CenterWatch Training Manuals and Directories

The Investigator's Guide to Clinical Research, 3rd edition
This 250-page step-by-step manual is filled with tips, instructions and insights for health professionals interested in conducting clinical trials. The *Investigator's Guide* is designed to help the novice clinical investigator get involved in conducting clinical trials. The guide is also a valuable resource for experienced investigative sites looking for ways to improve and increase their involvement and success in clinical research. Developed in accordance with ACCME, readers can apply for CME credits. An exam is provided online.

How to Find & Secure Clinical Grants
This 28-page guidebook is an ideal resource for healthcare professionals interested in conducting clinical trials. The guidebook provides tips and insights for new and experienced investigative sites to compete more effectively for clinical study grants.

How to Grow Your Investigative Site: A Guide to Operating and Expanding a Successful Clinical Research Center

This 300-page book is an ideal resource for clinical investigators interested in expanding their clinical trials operations in order to establish a more successful and effective research enterprise. Written by Barry Miskin, M.D., and Ann Neuer, the book is filled with practical case examples, insights, tips and reference resources designed to assist investigators and study personnel in growing a viable and successful clinical research business. Readers can apply for CME credits. An exam is provided online.

A Guide to Patient Recruitment:
Today's Best Practices and Proven Strategies

This 350-page manual is designed to help clinical research professionals improve the effectiveness of their patient recruitment efforts. Written by Diana Anderson, Ph.D., with contributions from 15 industry experts and thought leaders, this guide offers real world, practical recruitment strategies and tactics. It is considered an invaluable resource for educating professionals who manage and conduct clinical research about ways to plan and execute effective patient recruitment and retention efforts. Readers can apply for CME credits. An exam is provided online.

Protecting Study Volunteers in Research, 2nd edition
A Manual For Investigative Sites

The second edition of our top-selling manual has doubled in size to address current and emerging issues that are critical to our system of human subject protection oversight. *Protecting Study Volunteers in Research* is a suggested educational resource by NIH and FDA (source: NIH Notice OD-00-039, 2000, page 37841; Federal Registry 2002) and is designed to help organizations provide the highest standards of safe and ethical treatment of study volunteers. Written specifically for academic institutions and IRBs actively involved in clinical trials, the manual is also applicable to independent investigative sites. The book has been developed in accordance with the ACCME. Readers can apply for CME credits or Nursing Credit Hours. An exam is provided with each manual and is also available online.

The CRA's Guide to Monitoring Clinical Research

This 450+ page CE-accredited book is an ideal resource for novice and experienced CRAs, as well as professionals interested in pursuing a career as study monitors. The CRA's Guide covers important topics along with updated regulations, guidelines and worksheets, including resources such as: 21 CFR Parts 50, 54, 56 & 312 Guidelines, various checklists (monitoring visit, site evaluation, informed consent) and a study documentation file verification log. This manual will be routinely referenced throughout the CRA's career.

The New CenterWatch Drugs in Clinical Trials Database

The *Drugs in Clinical Trials Database* is a comprehensive web-based, searchable resource offering detailed profiles of new investigational treatments in phase I through III clinical trials. Updated daily, this online and searchable directory provides information on more than 2,000 drugs for more than 600 indications worldwide in a well-organized and easy-to-reference format. Detailed profile information is provided for each drug. A separate section is provided on pediatric treatments. The *Drugs in Clinical Trials Database* is an ideal online resource for industry professionals to use for monitoring the performance of drugs in clinical trials; tracking competitors' development activity; identifying development partners; and identifying clinical study grant opportunities.

The 2003 CenterWatch Directory of the Clinical Trials Industry

This comprehensive directory holds more than 1,000 pages of contact information and detailed company profiles for a wide range of organizations and individuals involved in the clinical trials industry. It is considered the authoritative reference resource for organizations involved in designing, managing, conducting and supporting clinical trials.

Profiles of Service Providers on the
CenterWatch Clinical Trials Listing Service™

The CenterWatch web site (www.centerwatch.com) attracts tens of thousands of sponsor and CRO company representatives every month that are looking for experienced service providers and investigative sites to manage and conduct their clinical trials. No registration is required. Sponsors and CROs use this online directory free of charge. The CenterWatch web site offers all contract service providers—both CROs and investigative sites—the opportunity to present more information than any other Internet-based service available. This service is an ideal way to secure new contracts and clinical study grants.

An Industry in Evolution

This 250-page sourcebook provides extensive data and facts documenting clinical trial industry trends and benchmarked practices. The material—charts, statistics and analytical reports—is presented in an easy-to-reference format. This important and valuable resource is used for developing business strategies and plans, for preparing presentations and for conducting business and market intelligence.

CenterWatch Compilation Reports Series

These topic specific reports provide comprehensive, in-depth features, original research and analyses and fact-based company/institution business and financial profiles. Reports are available on Site Management Organizations, Academic Medical Centers, and Contract Research Organizations. Spanning nearly five years of in-depth coverage and analyses, these reports provide valuable insights into company strategies, market dynamics and successful business practices. Ideal for business planning and for market intelligence/market research activities.

The CenterWatch Patient Education Series

As part of ongoing reforms in human subject protection oversight, institutional and independent IRBs and research centers are actively identifying educational programs and assessment mechanisms to use with their study volunteers. These initiatives are of particular interest among those IRBs that are applying for voluntary accreditation with the Association for the Accreditation of Human Research Protection Programs (AAHRPP) and the National Committee for Quality Assurance (NCQA). CenterWatch offers a variety of educational communications for use by IRB and clinical research professionals.

Informed Consent™: A Guide to the Risks and Benefits of Volunteering for Clinical Trials
This comprehensive 300-page reference resource is designed to assist patients and health consumers in understanding the clinical trial process and their rights and recourse as study volunteers. Based on extensive review and input from bioethicists, regulatory and industry experts, the guide provides facts, insights and case examples designed to assist individuals in making informed decisions about participating in clinical trials. The guide is an ideal educational reference that research and IRB professionals can use to review with their study volunteers, to address volunteer questions and concerns, and to further build relationships with the patient community. Professionals also refer to this guide for assistance in responding to the media.

Volunteering For a Clinical Trial
This easy-to-read, six-page patient education brochure is designed for research centers to provide consistent, professional and unbiased educational information for their potential clinical study subjects. The brochure is IRB approved and is used by sponsors, CROs and investigative sites to help set patient expectations about participating in clinical trials. *Volunteering for a Clinical Trial* can be distributed in a variety of ways including direct mailings to patients, displays in waiting rooms, or as handouts to guide discussions. The brochure can be customized with company logos and custom information.

A Word from Study Volunteers: Opinions and Experiences of Clinical Trial Participants
This straightforward and easy-to-read ten-page pamphlet reviews the results of a survey conducted among more than 1,200 clinical research volunteers. This brochure presents first-hand experiences from clinical trial volunteers.

It offers valuable insights for individuals interested in participating in a clinical trial. The brochure can be customized with company logos and custom information.

The CenterWatch Clinical Trials Listing Service™

Now in its seventh year of operation, *The CenterWatch Clinical Trials Listing Service™* provides the largest and most comprehensive listing of Industry- and Government-sponsored clinical trials on the Internet. In 2002, the CenterWatch web site—along with numerous coordinated online and print affiliations—is expected to reach more than 8 million Americans. *The CenterWatch Clinical Trials Listing Service™* provides an international listing of more than 42,000, ongoing and IRB-approved phase I–IV clinical trials.

CenterWatch Periodicals

CenterWatch

Our award-winning monthly newsletter provides pharmaceutical and biotechnology companies, CROs, SMOs, academic institutions, research centers and the investment community with in-depth business news and insights, feature articles on trends and clinical research practices, original market intelligence and analysis, as well as grant lead information for investigative sites.

CWWeekly

This weekly newsletter, available as a fax or in electronic format, reports on the top stories and breaking news in the clinical trials industry. Each week the newsletter includes business headlines, financial information, market intelligence, drug pipeline and clinical trial results.

JobWatch

This web-based resource at www.centerwatch.com, complemented by a print publication, provides comprehensive listings of career and educational opportunities in the clinical trials industry, including a searchable resume database service and online CE- and CME-accredited learning modules. Companies use *JobWatch* regularly to identify qualified clinical research professionals and career and educational services.

CenterWatch Intelligence Services

Market Intelligence Reports and Services

With nearly a decade of experience gathering original data and writing about all aspects of the clinical research enterprise, the *CenterWatch Market Intelligence Department* is uniquely positioned to provide a wide range of market research services designed to assist organizations in making more informed strategic business decisions that impact their clinical research activities. Our clients include major biopharmaceutical companies, CROs and contract service providers, site networks, investment analysts and management consulting firms. CenterWatch brings unprecedented industry knowledge, extensive industry-wide relationships and expertise gathering, analyzing and presenting primary and secondary quantitative and qualitative data. Along with our custom research projects for clients, CenterWatch also facilitates on-site management forums designed to explore critical business trends and their implications. These sessions offer a wealth of data and a unique opportunity for senior professionals to think about business problems in new ways.

TrialWatch Site-Identification Service

Several hundred sponsor and CRO companies use the TrialWatch service to identify prospective investigative sites to conduct their upcoming clinical trials. Every month, companies post bulletins of their phase I–IV development programs that are actively seeking clinical investigators. These bulletins are included in *CenterWatch*—our flagship monthly publication that reaches as many as 25,000 experienced investigators every month. Use of the *TrialWatch* service is FREE.

Content License Services

CenterWatch offers both database content and static text under license. All CenterWatch content can be seamlessly integrated into your company Internet, Intranet or Extranet web site(s) with or without frames. Our database offerings include: the *Clinical Trials Listing Service™*, *Clinical Trial Results, Drugs in Clinical Trials, Newly Approved Drugs, The Clinical Trial Industry Directory*, and *CW-Mobile* for Wireless OS® Devices. Our static text offerings include: an editorial feature on background information on clinical trials and a glossary of clinical trial terminology.